Cardiac Arrhythmias: A Compendium

Editor

OTTO COSTANTINI

MEDICAL CLINICS OF NORTH AMERICA

www.medical.theclinics.com

Consulting Editor
BIMAL H. ASHAR

September 2019 • Volume 103 • Number 5

ELSEVIER

1600 John F. Kennedy Boulevard • Suite 1800 • Philadelphia, Pennsylvania, 19103-2899

http://www.theclinics.com

MEDICAL CLINICS OF NORTH AMERICA Volume 103, Number 5
September 2019 ISSN 0025-7125, ISBN-13: 978-0-323-67858-2

Editor: Jessica McCool
Developmental Editor: Kristen Helm

Medical Clinics of North America (ISSN 0025-7125) is published bimonthly by Elsevier Inc., 360 Park Avenue South, New York, NY 10010-1710. Months of publication are January, March, May, July, September, and November. Business and editorial offices: 1600 John F. Kennedy Boulevard, Suite 1800, Philadelphia, PA 19103-2899. Periodicals postage paid at New York, NY, and additional mailing offices. Subscription prices are USD $284.00 per year (US individuals), $611.00 per year (US institutions), $100.00 per year (US Students), $353.00 per year (Canadian individuals), $794.00 per year (Canadian institutions), $200.00 per year (Canadian and foreign students), $406.00 per year (foreign individuals), and $794.00 per year (foreign institutions). To receive student/resident rate, orders must be accompanied by name of affiliated institution, date of term, and the signature of program/residency coordinator on institution letterhead. Orders will be billed at individual rate until proof of status is received. Foreign air speed delivery is included in all Clinics' subscription prices. All prices are subject to change without notice. **POSTMASTER:** Send address changes to *Medical Clinics of North America*, Elsevier Health Sciences Division, Subscription Customer Service, 3251 Riverport Lane, Maryland Heights, MO 63043. **Customer Service: Telephone: 1-800-654-2452** (U.S. and Canada); **1-314-447-8871** (outside U.S. and Canada). **Fax: 314-447-8029. E-mail: journalscustomerserviceusa@elsevier.com** (for print support); **journalsonlinesupport-usa@elsevier.com** (for online support).

Reprints. For copies of 100 or more of articles in this publication, please contact the Commercial Reprints Department, Elsevier Inc., 360 Park Avenue South, New York, NY 10010-1710. Tel.: 212-633-3874; Fax: 212-633-3820; E-mail: reprints@elsevier.com.

Medical Clinics of North America is also published in Spanish by McGraw-Hill Interamericana Editores S. A., P.O. Box 5-237, 06500 Mexico, D.F., Mexico.

Medical Clinics of North America is covered in *MEDLINE/PubMed (Index Medicus), Current Contents, ASCA, Excerpta Medica, Science Citation Index,* and *ISI/BIOMED*.

PROGRAM OBJECTIVE
The goal of the *Medical Clinics of North America* is to keep practicing physicians up to date with current clinical practice by providing timely articles reviewing the state of the art in patient care.

TARGET AUDIENCE
All practicing physicians and other healthcare professionals.

LEARNING OBJECTIVES
Upon completion of this activity, participants will be able to:
1. Review the pathophysiology, epidemiology, and risk factors of Sudden Cardiac Death (SCD), as well as treatment strategies for patients at risk for SCD.
2. Discuss key clinical concepts of cardiac electrophysiology.
3. Recognize risks and benefits of antiarrhythmic drugs.

ACCREDITATION
The Elsevier Office of Continuing Medical Education (EOCME) is accredited by the Accreditation Council for Continuing Medical Education (ACCME) to provide continuing medical education for physicians.

The EOCME designates this journal-based CME activity for a maximum of 14 *AMA PRA Category 1 Credit*(s)™. Physicians should claim only the credit commensurate with the extent of their participation in the activity.

All other healthcare professionals requesting continuing education credit for this enduring material will be issued a certificate of participation.

DISCLOSURE OF CONFLICTS OF INTEREST
The EOCME assesses conflict of interest with its instructors, faculty, planners, and other individuals who are in a position to control the content of CME activities. All relevant conflicts of interest that are identified are thoroughly vetted by EOCME for fair balance, scientific objectivity, and patient care recommendations. EOCME is committed to providing its learners with CME activities that promote improvements or quality in healthcare and not a specific proprietary business or a commercial interest.

The planning committee, staff, authors and editors listed below have identified no financial relationships or relationships to products or devices they or their spouse/life partner have with commercial interest related to the content of this CME activity:
Khaled Abozguia, MD,MRCP (London), PhD; Soufian T. AlMahameed, MD; Bimal H. Ashar, MD, MBA, FACP; Shajil Chalil, FRCP; Otto Costantini, MD; Vishal Dahya, MD; Noha Elbanhawy, MD, MRCP; Martin P. Emert, MD, FACC, FHRS; John Hornick, MD; Mohammad-Ali Jazayeri, MD; Gautham Kalahasty, MD; Alison Kemp; Jessica Kline, DO; Arun Umesh Mahtani, MBBS; Pranav Mankad, MD; Evan Martow, MDCM, BMSC; Jessica McCool; Viwe Mtwesi, MB ChB,FCP(SA); Devi Gopinath Nair, MD, FHRS; Kara J. Quan, MD, FACP, FACC, FHRS; Roopinder Sandhu, MD, MPH; Melanie M. Steffen, BSN; Jeyanthi Surendrakumar; Tyler L. Taigen, MD, FHRS; Ohad Ziv, MD.

The planning committee, staff, authors and editors listed below have identified financial relationships or relationships to products or devices they or their spouse/life partner have with commercial interest related to the content of this CME activity:
Guy Amit, MD, MPH: serves on a speakers bureau and/or is a consultant/advisor for Pfizer Inc and Bayer AG and receives research support from Servier

Michael J. Cutler, DO, PhD: is a consultant/advisor for Biosense Webster, Inc.

Jeffery S. Osborn, MD: serves on a speakers bureau and is a consultant/advisor for Abbott and Spectranetics

UNAPPROVED/OFF-LABEL USE DISCLOSURE
The EOCME requires CME faculty to disclose to the participants;
1. When products or procedures being discussed are off-label, unlabelled, experimental, and/or investigational (not US Food and Drug Administration [FDA] approved); and
2. Any limitations on the information presented, such as data that are preliminary or that represent ongoing research, interim analyses, and/or unsupported opinions. Faculty may discuss information about pharmaceutical agents that is outside of FDA-approved labelling. This information is intended solely for CME and is not intended to promote off-label use of these medications. If you have any questions, contact the medical affairs department of the manufacturer for the most recent prescribing information.

TO ENROLL

To enroll in the *Medical Clinics of North America* Continuing Medical Education program, call customer service at 1-800-654-2452 or sign up online at http://www.theclinics.com/home/cme. The CME program is available to subscribers for an additional annual fee of USD $300.90.

METHOD OF PARTICIPATION

In order to claim credit, participants must complete the following;
1. Complete enrolment as indicated above.
2. Read the activity.
3. Complete the CME Test and Evaluation. Participants must achieve a score of 70% on the test. All CME Tests and Evaluations must be completed online.

CME INQUIRIES/SPECIAL NEEDS

For all CME inquiries or special needs, please contact elsevierCME@elsevier.com.

Contributors

CONSULTING EDITOR

BIMAL H. ASHAR, MD, MBA, FACP
Associate Professor of Medicine, Division of General Internal Medicine, Johns Hopkins
School of Medicine, Baltimore, Maryland, USA

EDITOR

OTTO COSTANTINI, MD
Director, Clinical Research and Education, Associate Director, Cardiovascular Disease
Fellowship, Summa Health Heart and Vascular Institute, Summa Health System, Akron,
Ohio, USA

AUTHORS

KHALID ABOZGUIA, MD, MRCP (London), PhD
Director, Cardiac Electrophysiology Services, Consultant Cardiologist
Electrophysiologist, Lancashire Cardiac Center, Blackpool Victoria Hospital, Blackpool
Teaching Hospitals Foundation Trust, Blackpool, United Kingdom

SOUFIAN T. ALMAHAMEED, MD
Heart and Vascular Research Center, MetroHealth Campus of Case Western Reserve
University, Cleveland, Ohio, USA

GUY AMIT, MD, MPH
Cardiac Electrophysiology and Pacing, Division of Cardiology, Department of
Medicine, McMaster University, Hamilton General Hospital, Hamilton, Ontario,
Canada

SHAJIL CHALIL, FRCP
Head, Cardiology Department, Cardiac Electrophysiology Consultant, Lancashire Cardiac
Center, Blackpool Victoria Hospital, Blackpool Teaching Hospitals Foundation Trust,
Blackpool, United Kingdom

OTTO COSTANTINI, MD
Director, Clinical Research and Education, Associate Director, Cardiovascular Disease
Fellowship, Summa Health Heart and Vascular Institute, Summa Health System, Akron,
Ohio, USA

MICHAEL J. CUTLER, DO, PhD
Intermountain Heart Rhythm Specialist, Intermountain Medical Center, Murray, Utah,
USA

VISHAL DAHYA, MD
Cardiology Fellow, Cardiovascular Disease, Summa Health System, NEOMED University,
Akron City Hospital, Akron, Ohio, USA

NOHA ELBANHAWY, MD, MRCP
Cardiology Specialist Registrar, Lancashire Cardiac Center, Blackpool Teaching Hospitals, Blackpool, United Kingdom

MARTIN P. EMERT, MD, FACC, FHRS
Associate Professor, Medicine, Director, Ambulatory Cardiac Arrhythmia Device Services, Division of Electrophysiology, Department of Cardiovascular Medicine, University of Kansas Medical Center, Kansas City, Kansas, USA

JOHN HORNICK, MD
Cardiology Fellow, Cardiovascular Disease, Summa Health System, Akron, Ohio, USA

MOHAMMAD-ALI JAZAYERI, MD
Chief Fellow, Department of Cardiovascular Medicine, University of Kansas Medical Center, Kansas City, Kansas, USA

GAUTHAM KALAHASTY, MD
Program Director, Cardiovascular Disease Fellowship Program, Associate Professor, Medicine, Department of Electrophysiology, Virginia Commonwealth University Health System, Richmond, Virginia, USA

JESSICA KLINE, DO
Cardiovascular Disease Fellow, Summa Health Heart and Vascular Institute, Cardiology Fellow, Cardiovascular Disease, Summa Health System, Akron, Ohio, USA

ARUN UMESH MAHTANI, MBBS
Resident, Department of Cardiac Electrophysiology, St. Bernard's Heart and Vascular Center, Jonesboro, Arkansas, USA

PRANAV MANKAD, MD
Fellow, Cardiovascular Medicine, Department of Cardiology, Virginia Commonwealth University Health System, Richmond, Virginia, USA

EVAN MARTOW, BMSC, MDCM
Senior Resident, Division of Cardiology, University of Alberta, University of Alberta Hospital, Walter Mackenzie Health Sciences Centre, Edmonton, Alberta, Canada

VIWE MTWESI, MB ChB, FCP(SA)
Division of Cardiology, Department of Medicine, McMaster University, Hamilton General Hospital, Hamilton, Ontario, Canada

DEVI GOPINATH NAIR, MD, FHRS
Director, Department of Cardiac Electrophysiology, St. Bernard's Heart and Vascular Center, Jonesboro, Arkansas, USA

JEFFERY S. OSBORN, MD
Intermountain Heart Rhythm Specialist, Intermountain Medical Center, Murray, Utah, USA

KARA J. QUAN, MD, FACP, FACC, FHRS
Associate Professor, Medicine, Case Western Reserve University, Cleveland, Ohio, USA

ROOPINDER SANDHU, MD, MPH
Associate Professor, Division of Cardiology, University of Alberta, Walter Mackenzie Health Sciences Centre, Edmonton, Alberta, Canada

MELANIE M. STEFFEN, BSN
Intermountain Heart Rhythm Specialist, Intermountain Medical Center, Murray, Utah, USA

TYLER L. TAIGEN, MD, FHRS
Co-Director, Electrophysiology Laboratory, Section of Pacing and Electrophysiology, Department of Cardiovascular Medicine, Cleveland Clinic Foundation, Cleveland, Ohio, USA

OHAD ZIV, MD
Heart and Vascular Research Center, MetroHealth Campus of Case Western Reserve University, Cleveland, Ohio, USA

Contents

> This article represents an overview of the basic concepts of cardiac elec-trophysiology. This relatively new field became a subspecialty of cardiol-ogy in the mid-1990s due to the rapid development of equipment that allowed the study and cure of cardiac arrhythmias percutaneously. Simul-taneously, technology provided the field with percutaneous cardiac implantable electronic devices designed to protect patients from life-threatening bradyarrhythmias and tachyarrhythmias. Recently, the field has focused on the ablative treatment of atrial fibrillation, the most common arrhythmia facing an aging population, and the diagnosis and management of many inherited arrhythmias through advances in under-standing of their genetic cause.

> A 12-lead electrocardiogram (ECG) is the most commonly ordered cardiac test. Although data are not robust, guidelines recommend against per-forming an ECG in patients who are asymptomatic, even if they have a higher risk of developing cardiovascular disease in the long term. Conversely, patients with cardiac symptoms, including chest pain, dys-pnea, palpitation, and syncope, should have an ECG performed in the of-fice. Computerized algorithms exist ubiquitously to guide interpretation, but they can be the source of erroneous information. A stepwise approach is given to guide the primary care physician's approach to the systematic interpretation of ECG tracings.

> Palpitation is common. It is often accompanied by dizziness, lighthead-edness, near syncope, and even syncope. It may be difficult to confirm a diagnosis in patients with infrequent symptoms. Several tools are avail-able to document arrhythmias in the workup of a patient with palpitation, including 24-hour Holter monitoring, 30-day external continuous monitoring, and implantable loop recorders. A number of private com-panies are now able to empower patients to monitor heart rates and

even give accurate rhythm strips. This article reviews the current data on how to make the diagnosis and which tools to use in the primary care setting.

Cardiac arrhythmia is a common cause of syncope. The prompt identification of arrhythmic syncope has diagnostic and prognostic implications. In this article, an approach to identifying and managing arrhythmic syncope is discussed, including key findings from the history, physical examination, electrocardiogram, role of risk stratification, use of supplemental investigations, and treatment.

With recent advances in genetic diagnostics, many inherited diseases, which can cause life-threatening arrhythmias, are being better characterized. Many of these diseases are caused by genetic disorders that affect the function of the ion channels that regulate the action potential or the function of important cardiac muscle regulatory proteins. This article summarizes the diseases that we have learned about, such as the long QT syndrome, Brugada syndrome, and catecholaminergic polymorphic ventricular tachycardia. The article examines the diagnosis, genetic screening of patients and their relatives, management, and referral to a specialist for further therapy.

The narrow therapeutic window of antiarrhythmic drugs makes their use clinically challenging. A solid understanding of the mechanisms of arrhythmias and how antiarrhythmics affect these mechanisms is only a preliminary step in their appropriate selection. Clinical factors, side-effect profiles, and proarrhythmic risks are more important than the cellular mechanisms of actions in drug selection and monitoring. This article provides a simplified approach to understanding cellular mechanisms and provides a practical approach to the selection and use of this important class of medications.

Atrial fibrillation (AF) is the most common arrhythmia and its management may be organized into risk stratification and/or treatment of heart failure, stroke prevention, and symptom control. At the core of symptom control, treatment is tailored to either allow AF continue with controlled heart rates, so-called rate control, versus restoring and maintaining sinus rhythm or rhythm control. Rate control strategies mainly use rate-modulating medications, whereas rhythm control treatment includes therapy aimed at restoring sinus rhythm, including pharmacologic and direct current cardioversion, as well as maintenance of sinus rhythm, including antiarrhythmic medications and ablation therapy.

Oral anticoagulation significantly reduces the risk of stroke in patients with atrial fibrillation (AF), and the decision to initiate therapy is based on assessing the patient's yearly risk of stroke. Although warfarin remains the drug of choice in patients with AF and artificial mechanical valves, the novel anticoagulation agents are becoming the drug of choice for all other patients with AF, because of their efficacy, safety, and ease of use. This article summarizes the current evidence for stroke prevention in AF, including valvular AF, subclinical AF, AF in patients with renal insufficiency, as well as stroke prevention around AF cardioversion.

The term paroxysmal supraventricular tachycardia encompasses a heterogeneous group of arrhythmias with different electrophysiologic characteristics. Knowledge of the mechanism of each supraventricular tachycardia is important in determining management in the office, at the bedside, and in the electrophysiology laboratory. Paroxysmal supraventricular tachycardias have an abrupt onset and offset, typically initiating and terminating with premature atrial ectopic beats. In the acute setting, both vagal maneuvers and pharmacologic therapy can be effective in arrhythmia termination. Catheter ablation has revolutionized therapy for many supraventricular tachycardias, and newer techniques have significantly improved ablation efficacy and decreased periprocedural complications and procedure times.

Ventricular arrhythmias is commonly seen in medical practice. It may be completely benign or portend high risk for sudden cardiac death. Therefore, it is important that clinicians be familiar with and able to promptly recognize and manage ventricular arrhythmias when confronted with it clinically. In many cases, curative therapy for a given ventricular arrhythmia may be provided after a thorough understanding of the underlying substrate and mechanism. In this article, the authors broadly review the current classification of the different ventricular arrhythmias encountered in medical practice, provide brief background regarding the different mechanisms, and discuss practical diagnosis and management scenarios.

In this article, the authors review the different types of sinus node and atrioventricular node diseases that lead to bradyarrhythmias with their associated symptoms, the diagnostic investigations needed to assess

the degree of disease, and the therapeutic management, including the indications for permanent pacing.

Mohammad-Ali Jazayeri and Martin P. Emert

Sudden cardiac death (SCD) is a leading cause of death in the United
States. Despite improvements in therapy, the incidence of SCD as a proportion of overall cardiovascular death remains relatively unchanged. This
article aims to answer the question, "Who is at risk for SCD?" In the process, it reviews the definition, pathophysiology, epidemiology, and risk
factors of SCD. Patients at risk for SCD and appropriate treatment strategies are discussed.

Melanie M. Steffen, Jeffery S. Osborn, and Michael J. Cutler

Cardiac implantable electronic devices (CIEDs) provide lifesaving therapy
for the treatment of bradyarrhythmias, ventricular tachyarrhythmias, and
advanced systolic heart failure. Advances in CIED therapy have expanded
the number of patients receiving permanent pacemakers, implantable cardioverter defibrillators, and cardiac resynchronization therapy devices.
These devices improve quality of life and, in many cases, reduce mortality.
However, limitations remain in the management of patients who require
CIED therapy. This article provides a broad overview of CIED therapy in
the management of the cardiac patient.

Jessica Kline and Otto Costantini

Cardiac defects are the most common congenital defects, accounting for
approximately 9 per 1000 births. Patients with structural heart disease
related to congenital diseases are prone to develop intrinsic rhythm abnormalities as a result of altered physiology. In addition, they are at an
increased risk of developing acquired arrhythmias secondary to the nature
of surgical interventions done to improve physiologic function in the setting
of these defects. Arrhythmia management and risk stratification pose
particularly complex challenges to clinicians managing this population.

Foreword
Deviant Behavior

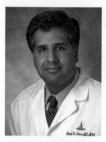

Bimal H. Ashar, MD, MBA, FACP
Consulting Editor

Constancy is something we perpetually search out in medicine. Patients seek medical care when there is a break from the feeling of constancy. Fatigue, insomnia, change in bowel habits, and heart palpitations are some of the most common complaints during a primary care visit. As providers, we inquire about "balanced" diets and "regular" exercise, and we seek out aberrant habits, such as cigarette and drug use and excess alcohol consumption. During the physical examination, we want to know if the "pupils are equal," bowel sounds are "normoactive," and whether the heart sounds are "regular rate and rhythm."

How we diagnose and treat aberrancies is what defines the practice of medicine. In 1930, Johns Hopkins University engineering student William Kouwenhoven invented a device intended to treat some of these aberrancies. He was able to externally jump start the heart in dogs. Several years later in 1947, surgeon Claude Beck successfully used such a device (defibrillator) in a human who survived a ventricular fibrillation arrest. Today, the public is encouraged to learn how to locate and use automated external defibrillators in order to maximize survival of patients with sudden cardiac death.

In this issue of the *Medical Clinics of North America*, my friend and colleague Dr Costantini has assembled a team of cardiologists who discuss the approach to diagnosis and treatment of cardiac arrhythmias. In most cases, correcting the anomaly may be the most appropriate course of action, especially given the advances in treatment

Med Clin N Am 103 (2019) xv–xvi
https://doi.org/10.1016/j.mcna.2019.05.010
0025-7125/19/© 2019 Published by Elsevier Inc.
medical.theclinics.com

modalities. However, some conditions may not require correction, just management and control of the deviant electrical behavior.

Bimal H. Ashar, MD, MBA, FACP
Division of General Internal Medicine
Johns Hopkins University
School of Medicine
601 North Caroline Street
#7143
Baltimore, MD 21287, USA

E-mail address:
Bashar1@jhmi.edu

Preface
Electricity 101: Simplifying the World of Rhythms and Devices

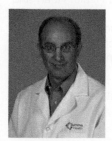

Otto Costantini, MD
Editor

Internists are faced daily with patients with symptoms related to either tachyarrhythmias or bradyarrhythmias. It can often be difficult to determine whether such conditions are benign or malignant. Palpitation, dizziness, syncope, shortness of breath, and even chest pain can be often traced back to common rhythm disorders. Some of the most common clinical diagnoses encompass rhythm disorders, such as atrial fibrillation, supraventricular tachycardia, sinus node dysfunction, premature ventricular contractions, and ventricular tachycardia, in patients with heart failure. The internist will often have the initial interaction with the patient, will need to know what testing to order, and will need to when to make a referral. The field of electrophysiology, a subspecialty of cardiology, emerged only 25 to 30 years ago. Over the last 3 decades, the diagnostic and therapeutic tools have grown exponentially thanks to a rapid evolution in technology for both devices and electrophysiologic equipment. From a diagnostic standpoint, the 24-hour Holter monitor is no longer standard of care for most rhythm diagnoses as better external monitors and even implanted monitors have been developed. In addition, invasive electrophysiologic studies are now available to diagnose and possibly treat many arrhythmias. From a therapeutic standpoint, antiarrhythmic medications, radiofrequency ablation, pacemakers to protect patients from bradycardias, defibrillators to protect patients from dangerous ventricular tachyarrhythmias, and cardiac resynchronization devices to improve left ventricular ejection fraction in patients with cardiomyopathy have progressed to the point where we can now offer a cure for many supraventricular rhythms and protection from life-threatening bradyarrhythmias and ventricular tachyarrhythmias. In this issue of the *Medical Clinics of North America*, we offer a compendium that simplifies the most common electrical problems encountered by the internist today. We cover all devices, their indication, their differences, and their complications. We cover the pharmacologic and nonpharmacologic management of supraventricular and ventricular arrhythmias. We cover the diagnosis

Med Clin N Am 103 (2019) xvii–xviii
https://doi.org/10.1016/j.mcna.2019.05.009
0025-7125/19/© 2019 Published by Elsevier Inc.

and management of bradyarrhythmias and when to be concerned that syncope is arrhythmic in nature. It is a comprehensive summary geared toward internists and designed to make internists more comfortable in diagnosing and managing conditions that, although common, can often be complicated. We hope that the readers will find this issue helpful and refer to it frequently as their "electricity" manual.

Otto Costantini, MD
Summa Health Heart and
Vascular Institute
Summa Health System
95 Arch Street Suite 350
Akron, OH 44304, USA

E-mail address:
costantinio@summahealth.org

Basic Principles of Cardiac Electrophysiology

Otto Costantini, MD

KEYWORDS

- Electrocardiography • Pacemakers and defibrillators
- Atrial and ventricular tachyarrhythmias • Atrial and ventricular bradyarrhythmias

KEY POINTS

- The field of cardiac electrophysiology is relatively new and has exploded due to rapid technological advances.
- Testing for electrophysiologic problems ranges from simple electrocardiograms, to implantable monitors, to complex invasive ablative procedures.
- Treatment of most atrial and ventricular arrhythmias can be curative via radiofrequency ablation.
- Devices have been instrumental in the management of patients with bradycardias, those at risk for ventricular tachyarrhythmias, and those with heart failure.
- The future will focus on the treatment of atrial fibrillation, the management of ventricular tachycardia, and the role of genetic testing for inherited cardiac arrhythmias.

INTRODUCTION

The field of clinical cardiac electrophysiology is a relatively new subspecialty of cardiology, as the first board certification was offered in 1994. The field evolved rapidly over the prior 25 years, ever since technology allowed for the percutaneous recordings of intracardiac electrograms. The first His bundle recording was obtained in 1969.[1] In the 1970s and 1980s, the field relied on percutaneous diagnosis of arrhythmias with the use of diagnostic catheters advanced into the right and left side of the heart via venous and arterial conduits, but treatment of arrhythmias, such as Wolff-Parkinson-White (WPW) pathways, atrial fibrillation, or ventricular tachycardia, was surgical.[2,3] In the late 1980s and 1990s, technological advances resulting in the development of catheters that could deliver first direct current shocks and subsequently safer radiofrequency ablation (RFA) led to the modern day practice of percutaneous catheter ablation for most atrial and ventricular tachyarrhythmias.[4,5]

Disclosure Statement: The author has no financial relationships to disclose pertaining to the content of this article.
Cardiovascular Disease Fellowship, Summa Health Heart and Vascular Institute, Summa Health System, 95 Arch Street, Suite 350, Akron, OH 44304, USA
E-mail address: costantinio@summahealth.org

Med Clin N Am 103 (2019) 767–774
https://doi.org/10.1016/j.mcna.2019.04.002
0025-7125/19/© 2019 Elsevier Inc. All rights reserved.

medical.theclinics.com

Almost simultaneously, devices to treat life-threatening bradyarrhythmias and tachyarrhythmias were being developed. The first pacemaker was implanted in 1958 for complete atrioventricular (AV) block.[6] Implantable defibrillators were initially developed in the 1980s and implanted surgically[7] until the advent of transvenous defibrillation leads and smaller generators allowed for prepectoral implantation in a fashion similar to modern pacemakers.

RADIOFREQUENCY ABLATION
Supraventricular Tachyarrhythmias

Supraventricular tachyarrhythmias are one of the most common problems encountered in the primary care settings. The patient can present to the office with self-terminating palpitation or with sustained, symptomatic tachyarrhythmias. The most common of these rhythms, and the one that has eluded an electrophysiologic cure, is atrial fibrillation. A whole article of this issue is dedicated to the diagnosis, differential diagnosis, and management of such rhythms. For the purposes of this introductory article, the author would like to highlight some key clinical concepts, as follows:

- The basic pathophysiologic mechanism of the overwhelming majority of such rhythms is reentry.[8] Reentry assumes the presence of 2 electrical pathways that have distinct electrophysiologic properties. One of the pathways conducts electricity slower than the other. The 2 pathways can be (A) Congenital: such as being born with an accessory pathway connecting the atrium and the ventricle (WPW) or being born with 2 pathways in the AV node (a "slow" and a "fast" pathway leading to AV nodal reentry tachycardia); (B) Aquired: such as in the case of an area of functional slow conduction/block in the atrium (typical atrial flutter) or an area of structural block, such as in the case of an atrial tachycardia around a scar created in the atrium after cardiac bypass surgery.
- Most of these arrhythmias are eminently curable, with a success rate in the 80% to 99% range depending on the type (**Table 1**). Because they often occur in a young healthy population, RFA has become the first-line therapy, rather than long-term medical treatment, in symptomatic patients with recurrent events.[9]

Table 1
Supraventricular arrhythmias and radiofrequency ablation

Arrhythmia Type	Amenable to RFA	Success Rate, %	Recurrence Rate, %	Site of RFA
AV nodal reentry	Yes	>95	<5	Slow pathway of AV node
Atrioventricular reentry (AP)	Yes	90–100	5–10	Accessory pathway (AP) RFA
Typical atrial flutter	Yes	95–100	5–10	Ablation line from TV to IVC
Unifocal atrial tachycardia	Yes	80–100	5–20	Right/left atrial tissue
Atypical atrial flutter	Yes	75–100	10–50	Right/left atrial tissue
Atrial fibrillation	Yes	50–100	20–50	Pulmonary veins/multiple atrial sites
Multifocal atrial tachycardia	No	—	—	—
Inappropriate sinus tachycardia	No	—	—	—

Abbreviations: AP, accessory pathway; IVC, inferior vena cava; TV, tricuspid valve.

- These arrhythmias are, for the most part, benign because they present typically with palpitation, dizziness, and shortness of breath, rather than with syncope. The only exception is the WPW syndrome, which can impart a small but real risk of sudden death.[10]

Atrial Fibrillation

Although atrial fibrillation is one of the supraventricular tachyarrhythmias, it deserves to be singled out in this article to make several key points, as follows:

- It is by far the most common rhythm encountered in clinical practice. Its prevalence is only due to the increase given an aging population and the many endemic risk factors that are associated with it, including hypertension, diabetes, sleep apnea, pulmonary disease, and structural heart disease. Just based on age alone, 5% to 10% of patients in their 70s will experience atrial fibrillation. That number increases to 10% to 20% in patients in their 80s.
- Although maintaining sinus rhythm is preferable in many patients, this remains the Holy Grail for today's practicing electrophysiologist. Medical treatment with the best antiarrhythmic drugs achieves sustained rhythm control only 50% to 60% of the time when the patient is followed for at least 1 year. Over longer follow-up periods, any antiarrhythmic drug is palliative, not curative, and significant side effects may occur with the most potent drugs.
- Although RFA offers the chance of a cure, and in some experts' opinion it should be considered first-line therapy in many patients, the success rates remain well below the ones established in other supraventricular arrhythmias, often necessitating multiple procedures.[11,12]
- The success rate of RFA is dependent on multiple variables. From an internist standpoint, it should be noted that even in expert centers, techniques are variable and controversy exists on where and how much atrial tissue to ablate or on what equipment to use. Pulmonary vein isolation is the mainstay of the RFA, but other parts of the left and right atrium are often ablated. Patient factors, such as the length of time that the patient has been in atrial fibrillation, the size and amount of scarring of the left and right atrium, and the presence of clinical risk factors like morbid obesity, also play a key role in the likelihood of a cure.[12]

Ventricular Tachyarrhythmias in Structurally Normal Hearts

Traditionally, ventricular tachyarrhythmias have been associated with a malignant prognosis. However, over the last 2 decades, several more benign conditions leading to frequent ventricular ectopy in the form of single premature ventricular contraction and even nonsustained and sustained episodes of ventricular tachycardia have been identified. Of these, the most commonly encountered rhythm is right ventricular outflow tachycardia. This rhythm is important to recognize because it can be ablated with good success, typically more than 80%.[13] Other rhythms are more uncommon. Unfortunately, even in structurally normal hearts, occasional malignant rhythms have been recognized. These occasional malignant rhythms are usually genetically based, and as the genetic diagnostic field has progressed, some can now be diagnosed with simple blood-based genetic testing.[14]

Ventricular Tachyarrhythmias in Structurally Abnormal Hearts

Patients with ischemic and nonischemic cardiomyopathies are at an increased risk of sudden cardiac death from ventricular tachycardia and ventricular fibrillation. These arrhythmias are also reentrant in mechanism, but the reentrant circuits are large, variable, and dynamic. They are dependent on areas of slow conduction that are present in the border zone of scars that are heterogeneous and related to areas of infarct in ischemic hearts, and fibrous scarring in nonischemic hearts. Because of the advent of implantable cardiac defibrillators, and because of the poor success rates in curing such arrhythmias, the role of RFA has been largely relegated to treating patients with frequent refractory episodes and recurrent defibrillator shocks.[15]

DEVICE THERAPY

Over the last half a century, the technology for device therapy has progressed as quickly, if not quicker, than the technology used for electrophysiologic studies and RFA. Cardiac-implantable electronic devices now are capable of protecting patients from bradyarrhythmias and ventricular tachyarrhythmias, and in select heart failure patients, can improve survival by providing biventricular (right and left ventricle) cardiac resynchronization therapy (CRT). **Table 2** shows the most common reasons for implanting pacemakers and defibrillators depending on the patient's clinical condition.[16,17]

DEVICE THERAPY FOR BRADYARRHYTHMIAS
Sinus Node Dysfunction

The definition and presentation of sinus node dysfunction are variable. The internist will be faced with many elderly patients who present with sinus bradycardia. However, in the absence of symptoms, this does not need to be treated. Typically, sinus node

Table 2
Device types based on clinical indications

Arrhythmia Type	Device Type	Number of Leads	Clinical Indications
Permanent atrial fibrillation with a slow ventricular response	Single-chamber ventricular pacemaker (VVI pacemaker)	1 RV lead	Symptomatic slow atrial fibrillation
Sinus node dysfunction or sick sinus syndrome with a preserved LVEF	Dual-chamber atrial and ventricular pacemaker (DDD pacemaker)	1 RA lead 1 RV lead	Symptomatic sinus bradycardia with or without atrial tachyarrhythmias
Symptomatic second- and third-degree AV block	Dual-chamber atrial and ventricular pacemaker (DDD pacemaker)	1 RA lead 1 RV lead	Symptomatic heart block with a preserved LVEF
Primary and secondary prevention of SCD with LVEF ≤35% and a *narrow QRS*	Dual-chamber atrial and ventricular defibrillator (DDD ICD)	1 RA lead 1 RV lead (pace/ defibrillate)	Ischemic and nonischemic cardiomyopathy, with or without prior VT/VF
Systolic heart failure with LVEF ≤35% and a *left bundle branch block*	Triple-chamber atrial, right and left ventricular defibrillator (CRT-D)	1 RA lead 1 RV lead (pace/ defibrillate) 1 LV lead	Symptomatic systolic heart failure *WITH* protection from SCD
Systolic heart failure with LVEF ≤35% and a *left bundle branch block*	Triple-chamber atrial, right and left ventricular pacemaker (CRT-P)	1 RA lead 1 RV lead *(PACE ONLY)* 1 LV lead	Symptomatic systolic heart failure *WITHOUT* protection from SCD

Abbreviations: LVEF, left ventricular ejection fraction; RA, right atrial; RV, right ventricular; SCD, sudden cardiac death; VF, ventricular fibrillation; VT, ventricular tachycardia.

dysfunction is thought secondary to senescence of the sinus node and presents in the seventh and eighth decade of life. Some key points are as follows:

- The symptoms of sinus node dysfunction can be striking, such as in those patients presenting with syncope due to long pauses, or much more subtle and difficult to ascertain, such as in those patients who present with exertional fatigue due to chronotropic incompetence.[18]
- A reversible cause is almost never present. Electrolyte abnormalities, especially in the presence of acute kidney injury, are the most common. In patients in whom drugs that cause sinus bradycardia are absolutely indicated for the treatment of other medical conditions, such as β-blockers postacute myocardial infarction or in heart failure, or antiarrhythmic drugs for the treatment of atrial fibrillation, a pacemaker is indicated to allow for continued appropriate drug treatment.[16]
- Sinus node dysfunction is the most common cause for needing device therapy, in the form of a dual-chamber pacemaker. In up to 50% of cases, it is associated with the presence of paroxysmal or persistent atrial tachyarrhythmias, most commonly atrial fibrillation. Together, the atrial bradyarrhythmias and tachyarrhythmias constitute the sick sinus syndrome.

Atrioventricular Node Dysfunction/Atrioventricular Block

Acquired AV block is the second most common reason for needing a pacemaker. AV block, too, like sinus node dysfunction, is typically a disease of the elderly, related to progressive fibrosis and degeneration of the AV node and the specialized His-Purkinjie conduction system. Of note:

- Reversible causes include electrolyte abnormalities, ischemia (rarely), or high vagal tone. Recurrent vagal syncope with prolonged AV block may be at times helped by pacing.[16] In a young person, infiltrative diseases, such as sarcoidosis, should be suspected. First-degree AV block is not an indication for pacing. Symptomatic second-degree and third-degree AV block are clear indications for pacing.
- The internist will often see elderly patients who are asymptomatic, but have clear electrocardiographic evidence of conduction disease. The most concerning of these are patients with trifascicular block. This is defined by a first-degree AV block, a right bundle branch block, and a left fascicular block (either the left anterior or the left posterior fascicle). Although asymptomatic patients have a higher than average chance to progress to high-degree AV block, the rate of progression is slow.[19,20] Therefore, such patients do not require pacing. On the other hand, patients with the electrocardiographic abnormalities described above who develop brief, transient dizzy spells or unexplained syncopal events almost surely have episodes of transient AV block and require pacing, even if no documentation can be made of the arrhythmia.[16]
- Transient dizziness and unexplained syncope in the elderly are typically cardiac in nature. The 2 most common reasons are orthostatic, dysautonomic hypotension, and transient bradyarrhythmias. Embarking on an expensive neurologic workup is often fruitless. In contrast, cardiac monitoring with an external 30-day event recorder, or in select cases with an internal loop recorder, can often lead to a diagnosis.[21]

DEVICE THERAPY FOR TACHYARRHYTHMIAS AND THE RISK OF SUDDEN CARDIAC DEATH

With the advent of the internal cardiac defibrillator (ICD) in the mid-1980s, incredible strides have been made in the prevention of sudden cardiac death.

Up until the early 1990s, these devices had to be implanted surgically, with a thoracotomy, and were reserved for patients who were lucky enough to have survived a cardiac arrest. In the late 1990s/early 2000s, large, well-designed, randomized, multicenter trials proved that the ICD improved survival compared with medical therapy alone in patients with both ischemic and nonischemic cardiomyopathy and an ejection fraction ≤35%, who had not yet suffered a ventricular tachyarrhythmic event.[22–25]

Most patients who are receiving ICDs today are getting them for primary prophylaxis of sudden death. As such, they typically only need a single-chamber right-ventricular ICD. However, many of these patients will have an atrial lead implanted to better discriminate between atrial and ventricular tachyarrhythmias and decrease the likelihood of inappropriate shocks from rapid atrial tachyarrhythmias like atrial fibrillation and atrial tachycardia.

The likelihood of a sudden death event with a device in place is extremely low. Most of these patients will progress to end-stage heart failure. The decision of when to turn the device off is a difficult one, and one that should be shared with patients and their family.[26]

For patients who experience recurrent, appropriate ICD shocks, the palliative role of drugs versus RFA is debated. Either provides only the small benefit of reducing the frequency of events, especially in elderly patients with advanced systolic heart failure. In select patients, a RFA can be curative.[27]

DEVICE THERAPY FOR HEART FAILURE

In addition to receiving the above described ICD, a subset of patients are candidates for a device that has been shown to improve heart failure symptoms and total mortality. Approximately 20% to 30% of patients with an ischemic or nonischemic cardiomyopathy have evidence of dyssynchrony between the ventricular septum and the lateral wall of the left ventricle, 1 wall contracting much sooner than the other. Such dyssynchrony causes decreased stroke volume, increased mitral valve regurgitation, and worsening heart failure. Such dyssynchrony is manifested best by a left bundle branch block on the electrocardiogram. The longer the QRS is on the electrocardiogram, the worse the dyssynchrony. By adding a left ventricular pacing lead to the right ventricular lead, the 2 walls contract more simultaneously, essentially "resynchronizing" the ventricular septum and the lateral wall of the left ventricle. This "resynchronization" is the pathophysiologic basis for improved symptoms, increased stroke volume and cardiac output, and decreased mitral valve regurgitation. Patients with a left ventricular ejection fraction ≤35%, a left bundle branch block with a QRS duration of more than 130 ms, and class II or III heart failure symptoms are candidates for these devices commonly referred to as biventricular ICDs or cardiac resynchronization therapy defibrillators (CRT-D).[28] Patients with right bundle branch block may also benefit from such devices, although the literature is more controversial. Finally, elderly patients who are candidates for a CRT device may want to forgo the protection from sudden cardiac death provided by a defibrillator, yet may still want to improve their quality of life and heart failure symptoms. Such patients are candidates for a CRT pacemaker (CRT-P) (see **Table 2**).

SUMMARY

In this introductory article, the authors illustrated, in broad strokes, the advances in electrophysiology over the last half century. They have found ways to cure most atrial tachyarrhythmias with RFA.[29] They have found ways to protect patients from dangerous, life-threatening bradyarrhythmias and ventricular tachyarrhythmias with cardiac implantable devices.[30,31] In the future, atrial fibrillation ablation will become more mainstream, and it is hoped, more successful at permanently curing the rhythm. At the same time, it is hoped advances in understanding the genetic basis of disease and in genetic testing will allow the diagnosis and prevention many of these disease processes before they even develop.

REFERENCES

1. Scherlag BJ, Lau SH, Helfant RH, et al. Catheter technique for recording His bundle activity in man. Circulation 1969;39:13–8.
2. Fischell TA, Stinson EB, Derby GC, et al. Long-term follow-up after surgical correction of Wolff-Parkinson-White syndrome. J Am Coll Cardiol 1987;9:283–7.
3. Cox JL, Schuessler RB, D'Agostino HJ Jr, et al. The surgical treatment of atrial fibrillation. III. Development of a definitive surgical procedure. J Thorac Cardiovasc Surg 1991;101:569–83.
4. Newman D, Evans GT Jr, Scheinman MM. Catheter ablation of cardiac arrhythmias. Curr Probl Cardiol 1989;14:117–64.
5. Morady F. Radio-frequency ablation as treatment for cardiac arrhythmias. N Engl J Med 1999;340:534–44.
6. Weirich WL, Gott VL, Lillehei CW. The treatment of complete heart block by the combined use of a myocardial electrode and an artificial pacemaker. Surg Forum 1958;8:360–3.
7. Mirowski M. The automatic implantable cardioverter-defibrillator: an overview. J Am Coll Cardiol 1985;6:461–6.
8. Tse G. Mechanisms of cardiac arrhythmias. J Arrhythmia 2016;32:75–81.
9. Richard L, Page MD, José A, et al. 2015 ACC/AHA/HRS guideline for the management of adult patients with supraventricular tachycardia. J Am Coll Cardiol 2016;67:e27–115.
10. Al-Khatib SM, Arshad A, Balk EM, et al. Risk stratification for arrhythmic events in patients with asymptomatic pre-excitation: a systematic review. Heart Rhythm 2016;13:e222–37.
11. Andrade JG, Verma A, Mitchell LB, et al, CCS Atrial Fibrillation Guidelines Committee. 2018 focused update of the Canadian Cardiovascular Society guidelines for the management of atrial fibrillation. Can J Cardiol 2018;34:1371–92.
12. January CT, Wann LS, Calkins H, et al. 2019 AHA/ACC/HRS focused update of the 2014 AHA/ACC/HRS guideline for the management of patients with atrial fibrillation. J Am Coll Cardiol 2019;74:104–32.
13. Latif S, Dixit S, Callans DJ. Ventricular arrhythmias in normal hearts. Cardiol Clin 2008;26:367–80.
14. Vatta M, Spoonamore KG. Use of genetic testing to identify sudden cardiac death syndromes. Trends Cardiovasc Med 2015;25:738–48.
15. Al-Khatib SM, Stevenson WG, Ackerman MJ, et al. 2017 AHA/ACC/HRS guideline for management of patients with ventricular arrhythmias and the prevention of sudden cardiac death. J Am Coll Cardiol 2018;72:e91–220.
16. Tracy CM, Epstein AE, Darbar D, et al. 2012 ACCF/AHA/HRS focused update incorporated into the ACCF/AHA/HRS 2008 guidelines for device-based therapy of cardiac rhythm abnormalities. JACC 2013;61:e6–75.
17. Gillis AM, Russo AM, Ellenbogen KA, et al. HRS/ACCF expert consensus statement on pacemaker device and mode selection. JACC 2012;60:682–703.
18. Mangrum JM, DiMarco JP. The evaluation and management of bradycardia. N Engl J Med 2000;342:703–9.

19. McAnulty JH, Rahimtoola SH, Murphy E, et al. Natural history of "high-risk" bundle-branch block: final report of a prospective study. N Engl J Med 1982; 307:137–43.
20. Fisch GR, Zipes DP, Fisch C. Bundle branch block and sudden death. Prog Cardiovasc Dis 1980;23:187–224.
21. Shen WK, Sheldon RS, Benditt DG, et al. 2017 ACC/AHA/HRS guideline for the evaluation and management of patients with syncope. Heart Rhythm 2017;14: e155–217.
22. Bardy GH, Lee KL, Mark DB, et al. Amiodarone or an implantable cardioverter-defibrillator for congestive heart failure. N Engl J Med 2005;352:225–37.
23. Buxton AE, Lee KL, Fisher JD, et al. A randomized study of the prevention of sudden death in patients with coronary artery disease. Multicenter Unsustained Tachycardia Trial Investigators. N Engl J Med 1999;341:1882–90.
24. Moss AJ, Hall WJ, Cannom DS, et al. Improved survival with an implanted defibrillator in patients with coronary disease at high risk for ventricular arrhythmia. Multicenter Automatic Defibrillator Implantation Trial Investigators. N Engl J Med 1996; 335:1933–40.
25. Moss AJ, Zareba W, Hall WJ, et al. Prophylactic implantation of a defibrillator in patients with myocardial infarction and reduced ejection fraction. N Engl J Med 2002;346:877–83.
26. Khera R, Pandey A, Link MS, et al. Managing implantable cardioverter-defibrillators at end-of-life: practical challenges and care considerations. Am J Med Sci 2019;357(2):143–50.
27. Sapp JL, Wells GA, Parkash R, et al. Ventricular tachycardia ablation versus escalation of antiarrhythmic drugs. N Engl J Med 2016;375:111–21.
28. Exner DV, Birnie DH, Moe G, et al. Canadian Cardiovascular Society guidelines on the use of cardiac resynchronization therapy: evidence and patient selection. Can J Cardiol 2013;29:182–95.
29. Andrade JG, Rivard L, Macle L. The past, the present, and the future of cardiac arrhythmia ablation. Can J Cardiol 2014;30:S431–41.
30. Luderitz B. Historical perspectives of cardiac electrophysiology. Hellenic J Cardiol 2009;50:3–16.
31. Mitrani RD, Myerburg RJ. Ten advances defining sudden cardiac death. Trends Cardiovasc Med 2016;26:23–33.

The Electrocardiogram
Still a Useful Tool in the Primary Care Office

John Hornick, MD[a], Otto Costantini, MD[b],*

KEYWORDS

- Electrocardiogram indications • Electrocardiogram interpretation
- Computerized ECG algorithms • Chronic heart disease • Chest pain evaluation
- Preoperative evaluation

KEY POINTS

- Indications for performing an electrocardiogram (ECG) in asymptomatic patients are rare.
- An ECG is indicated in patients with symptoms suggestive of cardiac disease.
- ECG interpretation should not rely solely on computerized algorithms, which can be erroneous.
- A systematic approach to interpreting an ECG is required to acquire all the appropriate information.

INTRODUCTION

In the evaluation of a patient with cardiac symptoms, the 12-lead electrocardiogram (ECG) is one of the simplest and easiest tests a primary care physician can obtain in the office. This simple test can help in any patient presenting with chest pain, shortness of breath, palpitations, or syncope. The ECG can also help in patients at risk for developing cardiac disease from chronic conditions, such as those with diabetes or long-standing hypertension. This article focuses on when and whether to obtain this test, how to interpret it, and how to determine whether an abnormal ECG should lead to referral to a cardiologist.

INDICATIONS FOR ORDERING AN AMBULATORY ELECTROCARDIOGRAM
Asymptomatic Patients

Screening electrocardiograms for asymptomatic patients
The usefulness of using an ECG as a screening tool to detect early cardiovascular disease (CVD) is controversial. Although epidemiologic studies in the 1980s suggest a

Disclosure Statement: The authors have no financial relationships to disclose pertaining to the content of this article.
[a] Cardiovascular Disease, Summa Health System, 95 Arch Street, Suite 300, Akron, OH 44304, USA; [b] Cardiovascular Disease Fellowship, Summa Health Heart and Vascular Institute, Summa Health System, 95 Arch Street, Suite 350, Akron, OH 44304, USA
* Corresponding author.
E-mail address: costantinio@summahealth.org

Med Clin N Am 103 (2019) 775–784
https://doi.org/10.1016/j.mcna.2019.04.003
0025-7125/19/© 2019 Elsevier Inc. All rights reserved.

medical.theclinics.com

higher risk of developing cardiac pathologic condition in patients with ECG abnormalities, such as right or left bundle branch block (RBBB or LBBB),[1,2] the prevalence of such abnormalities is low, in the order of 2% to 10%, even in patients with advanced age.[3] Therefore, because of the lack of data supporting its use, the current US Preventative Services Task Force (USPSTF) recommends against screening asymptomatic patients with a 12-lead ECG or an exercise ECG (recommendation level D, meaning the evidence suggests no net benefit, potential harm).[4] This recommendation applies to patients without CVD, defined as the presence of atherosclerosis manifested by prior coronary artery disease, stroke, or peripheral arterial disease, and at low risk of developing it. The likelihood for harm resulting from unnecessary testing outweighed the benefit of screening such low-risk individuals. Whether to screen asymptomatic patients without a CVD at moderate to high risk for developing it is more controversial. The USPSTF guidelines give it a level I recommendation, meaning the evidence is insufficient to make a recommendation. Such moderate- to high-risk patients benefit more from aggressive risk factor modification than from ECG screening. The USPSTF similarly offered recommendations against routine ECG screening for atrial fibrillation in asymptomatic patients unless pulse examination suggests an abnormality, such as an irregular rate or unexplained tachycardia.[5]

Special populations
Special populations with high-risk occupations in whom an acute cardiac event could potentially endanger others should be screened, although how often to screen is unknown. Hazardous occupations include heavy machinery operators, airline pilots, and commercial truck drivers.

Preparticipation/competition electrocardiograms in athletes
Whether to perform a screening ECG as part of the precompetition workup in both recreational and professional athletes has become a controversial topic over the last decade. In some European countries, young athletes are required to receive ambulatory ECGs before participating in sports, but screening programs are not uniform. A large trial screening adolescent soccer players in the United Kingdom was recently published.[6] It showed that among 11,168 patients screened with a program that included a health questionnaire, a physical examination, an ECG, and echocardiography, only 0.38% were found to have diseases associated with sudden cardiac death. The actual incidence of sudden cardiac death was 6.8 per 100,000 athletes. Most deaths occurred in patients who developed cardiomyopathies during follow-up and therefore were not identified during the screening ECG or echocardiogram. For the average "weekend warrior" athlete examined in an outpatient office, a risk versus benefit discussion should be considered before performing an outpatient ECG, because the ECG may result in potentially unnecessary follow-up testing and in holding an otherwise healthy individual from playing sports. In general, a preparticipation sports physical examination should only include a thorough history and physical examination, and importantly, a detailed review of a family history.

Preoperative evaluation
The purpose of a preoperative evaluation is to estimate the level of cardiac risk in a given noncardiac procedure as well as to identify potential areas for intervention to help decrease that risk. Several societal guidelines have been published over the years, including the 2014 American College of Cardiology/American Heart Association (ACC/AHA) guidelines on Perioperative Cardiovascular Evaluation and Care for Noncardiac Surgery.[7-10] The guidelines recommend that patients undergo an ECG (class I) if

- They have at least 1 risk factor for cardiac disease and are undergoing a vascular procedure
- They have known coronary artery disease, peripheral arterial disease, or stroke, and they are undergoing an intermediate or high-risk procedure

An ECG may be beneficial, although the data are not as clear, for patients without cardiac risk factors undergoing a vascular procedure (class IIA) or for those with at least 1 cardiac risk factor undergoing an intermediate-risk procedure (class IIB). On the other hand, an ECG is not indicated in asymptomatic patients undergoing low-risk procedures (class III). For such patients, a thorough history and physical examination should be sufficient in determining cardiac risk.

Symptomatic Patients

Patients may present to the office with a multitude of symptoms that could be cardiac. An ECG is typically indicated for symptoms of chest pain, palpitation, new dyspnea, or syncope.

Presenting symptom of chest pain

A routine office ECG is indicated in patients who describe previous or current chest pain to diagnose or help rule out life-threatening coronary syndromes.

- *ST segment elevation or ST segment depression of ≥1 mm* in 2 contiguous leads should raise the suspicion of an acute coronary syndrome. ST elevations always suggest an acute injury ST elevation myocardial infarction (STEMI), whereas ST depressions can indicate an acute injury (non-STEMI) or acute ischemia (ie, unstable angina). Regardless, these patients should be immediately referred to an emergency department (ED). If available in the office, patients should receive an aspirin and a sublingual nitroglycerin tablet × 3 every 5 minutes for symptom relief.
- *T-wave inversions* are more difficult to interpret and often require comparison to an old ECG, if available. Particular attention should be paid to T-wave inversions that are new. In a patient with active chest pain, new T-wave inversions often indicate acute ischemia and should be treated similarly to patients with ST segment depressions. However, inverted T waves can be chronic and typically related to an old infarct or long-standing hypertension with left ventricular hypertrophy (LVH).
- *The presence of Q waves* (initial negative deflection of the QRS complex, lasting at least 0.04 seconds or 1 small block in duration, or one-third the amplitude of the QRS complex) in 2 contiguous leads typically signifies a previous infarction. This finding is fairly nonspecific, however, and unless the patient is having active symptoms, no acute management is required. In such patients, it may be reasonable for the primary care physician to obtain an echocardiogram to assess for wall motion abnormalities in the coronary territory where the Q waves are seen. In addition, if the symptoms warrant it, these patients may benefit from stress testing or invasive coronary angiography.
- *Bundle branch blocks:* Bundle branch blocks are caused by an electrical abnormality of the His-Purkinje system of specialized ventricular conduction tissue. In an RBBB, right ventricular depolarization is delayed. In an LBBB, left ventricular depolarization is delayed. As a result, with both, the QRS duration is ≥120 milliseconds. On the ECG, the difference between the two is most manifest in the precordial leads. In an RBBB, the QRS has an RSR′ complex in V1 and V2, with a broad, deep S wave in V5 and V6. In an LBBB, there usually is a deep

S wave in V1 and V2, with a broad R wave in V5 and V6. In the setting of chest pain, a new LBBB (or presumed new if an old ECG is unavailable) has previously been described as an STEMI equivalent. Therefore, it should always be evaluated and treated as an acute coronary syndrome, even though it does not always represent an acute coronary occlusion. An LBBB causes the left ventricle to be depolarized and repolarized abnormally. As a result, electrocardiographic criteria for assessing for injury are grossly different.[11] Because in patients with an RBBB the left ventricle is depolarized normally, the ECG remains interpretable, and the criteria to assess for ischemia and injury patterns are unchanged from those in a normal ECG.

Presenting symptom of shortness of breath or palpitation

Although the causes of shortness of breath can be many, it can sometimes represent an anginal equivalent. It can occasionally produce ischemic changes similar to those listed in the chest pain section. If any of the ECG findings previously described are seen in a patient with acute shortness of breath, they should be treated as an anginal equivalent. Some of the most important ECG findings seen in patients with shortness of breath or palpitation include the following:

- *Sinus tachycardia* can be seen in multiple disorders and disease states. It does not always indicate an acute cardiac or pulmonary event, but it should alert the primary physician to an underlying pathologic process. Noncardiac causes, such as infections, anemia, dehydration, and chronic obstructive pulmonary disease exacerbations, should be considered. An acute pulmonary embolism (PE) is always in the differential. If a new murmur is detected, an acute or subacute valvular problem should be suspected. New edema or leg swelling, orthopnea, and paroxysmal nocturnal dyspnea suggest acute heart failure, systolic or diastolic. A chest radiograph is extremely helpful in these cases, in addition to the ECG. Depending on the hemodynamic stability of the patient and the acuity of the symptoms, these patients should be considered for echocardiography, occasionally on an urgent or emergent basis. In patients presenting with a PE, the most common ECG finding, is sinus tachycardia with a prominent S wave in lead I as well as a Q wave and isolated inverted T wave in lead III (S1Q3T3 sign). If a PE is suspected and the patient is symptomatic, the patient should be referred to the ED.
- *Atrial tachyarrhythmias* are a common ECG finding in patients presenting with dyspnea or palpitation. The most common of these are atrial fibrillation and atrial flutter. Other supraventricular tachycardias (SVTs) include atrial tachycardia and atrioventricular (AV) nodal reentry tachycardias. It should be noted that rarely is the rate of these tachycardias fast enough to cause syncope or near syncope. These are discussed in detail in other articles in this issue. From an ECG standpoint, the differential diagnosis is covered in detail in the 2015 ACC/AHA/Heart Rhythm Society guidelines for the management of SVT.[12]

Presenting symptom of lightheadedness, dizziness, or syncope

Obtaining an initial office ECG in patients presenting with lightheadedness, dizziness, presyncope, or syncope is absolutely indicated. It is not uncommon for such patients to have ECG abnormalities such as bradycardia or other forms of conduction disease responsible for the symptoms. In fact, hypotension, bradycardias, and, less often, tachycardias are more likely to cause these symptoms than a neurologic cause. In these cases, the ECG should be examined for the intrinsic heart rate (HR), the presence of P waves, the PR interval duration, the QRS interval duration, and the evidence that a QRS complex follows every P wave. The most common diagnoses causing these symptoms are as follows:

- *Sinus node dysfunction.* As the conduction system ages, the sinus node becomes sluggish. These patients will frequently present with HRs in the 40- to 50-beats-per-minute (bpm) range in the absence of drugs that can slow the sinus node. They will present with dizziness or presyncope and progressively worsening dyspnea on exertion and fatigue. The AV node and the His-Purkinje system are generally intact, and therefore, the QRS is narrow. AV nodal blocking agents, such as β-blockers and calcium channel blockers, should be decreased or discontinued entirely, although they are rarely the only primary cause. Patients with syncope may have sinus pauses lasting ≥5 seconds. When the symptoms are subtle, a stress ECG may help in diagnosing chronotropic incompetence. If the HR does not appropriately increase with exercise, the patient should be considered for permanent pacemaker implantation. A 24-hour Holter monitor or a 30-day event recorder may be very useful as well.
- *AV node disease:* AV nodal block on an ECG is not uncommon especially in patients who are older or have a long history of hypertension or coronary disease.
  - *First-degree AV block* is seen when the PR interval is longer than 200 milliseconds, and every P wave is followed by a QRS. By itself, it is not concerning, because it is only a sign of slow conduction through the atrial tissue. However, in conjunction with a QRS ≥120 milliseconds, it can indicate significant conduction disease. Patients with a long PR interval, an RBBB, and a left anterior or left posterior hemiblock have "trifascicular block." In this setting, patients with symptoms of near syncope or syncope frequently have, or slowly progress to, a higher-degree AV block. Therefore, they should be evaluated by an electrophysiologist for possible permanent pacemaker placement.
  - *Second-degree AV block* is characterized by the fact that not every P wave is followed by a QRS complex. Mobitz type I second-degree AV block, also known as Wenckebach AV block, occurs when there is progressive lengthening of the PR interval until a QRS is finally dropped. Mobitz type II occurs when QRS complexes are dropped without apparent PR interval prolongation. Of the 2 types of second-degree AV block, Mobitz type II is more likely to indicate significant His-Purkinje conduction disease. As a result, it is more likely to be present in the setting of a wide, prolonged QRS, and it is more likely to progress to third-degree/complete AV block. On the other hand, Mobitz type I AV block is more likely related to disease in the AV node itself and typically presents with a narrow QRS complex. That said, when symptomatic, all of these patients should be evaluated by an electrophysiologist because the likelihood is that they will need a pacemaker.
  - *Third-degree (complete) AV block* is characterized by the absence of any association between the P-to-P and QRS-to-QRS intervals, which are both marching at separate rates. If an office ECG shows complete AV block, the patient should be referred to the ED immediately because these rhythms are not always stable and could lead to sudden death.

INTERPRETATION OF A 12-LEAD ELECTROCARDIOGRAM
Can the Electrocardiogram Computer Algorithm Interpretation be Trusted?

Most ECGs are interpreted by noncardiologists. Knowing the basics of interpretation of an ECG can diagnose life-threatening cardiac events, screen for common arrhythmias, and determine which patients should be sent for evaluation by a cardiologist.

To help with ECG interpretation, proprietary computer algorithms have been developed by most manufacturers to give an immediate interpretation, a sort of "second opinion." The accuracy of these algorithms has improved over time, but it is still not as good as that of an expert reader. Computer interpretations were incorrect most frequently in arrhythmias, conduction disorders, and the diagnosis of pacemaker rhythms.[13] A study in 2012 suggested that although the positive predictive valve of a computer interpretation for normal sinus rhythm is high, atrial fibrillation was misdiagnosed 11.3% of the time.[14] Artifacts on the ECG can significantly decrease the accuracy of the computer read. For this reason, the computer read is helpful as a reference, but it is important for the provider to be proficient in the interpretation of the ECG.

APPROACH TO INTERPRETING AN ELECTROCARDIOGRAM

Guidelines exist for the performance and interpretation of a 12-lead ECG.[15–18] In addition, several books have been published to aid in ECG interpretation.[19,20] To help ensure important information is not missed, reading an ECG should be done in a stepwise fashion whereby every element of the ECG is observed sequentially. There are multiple approaches to this. It is important for each provider to have a systematic way of approaching the ECG. Here, the authors offer 1 such approach.

Step 1: Is the Electrocardiogram Interpretable?

It is important to make sure that the ECG is of the correct patient and that the scale and the speed of the tracing are appropriate. This function is a programmable function of the ECG machine. On the side of the ECG tracing, a small box will indicate the standard scale, which should be 1 mV/10 mm tall. When the scale is set to a different standard, the ECG may overestimate or underestimate the QRS amplitude or the ST segment changes. Similarly, if the speed is too slow or too fast (standard is 25 mm/s), the ECG tracing will be distorted. Standardization of lead placement and patient position are also important for longitudinal studies. The level of artifact should be low. Care should be taken to have the patient lie still and have good contact on the electrodes/skin interface, and one should make sure that the leads are placed in the correct configuration. Lead reversals are one of the most common reasons for erroneous interpretations.

Step 2: What Is the Heart Rate?

The computer algorithms are fairly accurate at determining HRs. However, determining an HR is straightforward. On the x-axis of the tracing, 1 small 1-mm box equals 0.04 seconds; a large box (5 small boxes) equals 0.2 seconds, and 5 large boxes equal 1 second. A standard ECG shows 10 seconds of data. If the rhythm is regular, the HR can be estimated by counting the number of big boxes between QRS complexes and dividing the number into 60 seconds to get a bpm rate. For example, if there is only 1 large box between QRS complexes (ie, 0.2 seconds), then 60/0.2 will give a HR of 300 bpm. A simple mnemonic is to remember that 1 big box between QRS complexes equals 300 bpm, 2 big boxes equal 150 bpm (60/0.4), 3 big boxes equal 100 bpm (60/0.6), 4 big boxes equal 75 bpm (60/0.8), and 5 big boxes equal 60 bpm (60/1.0). The simplest way to estimate the HR, if the rhythm is irregular, is to count the total number of QRS complexes seen on the rhythm strip. Multiplying this number by 6 will give the HR in beats per minute. This method is particularly useful in atrial fibrillation. A normal resting HR for an adult is 60 to 100 bpm. A tachycardia is a HR ≥100 bpm, whereas a bradycardia is a HR ≤60 bpm.

Step 3: What Is the Rhythm?

Sinus rhythm is a regular rhythm with P waves that are morphologically positive in the inferior leads (II, III, aVF). When the patient's rhythm is not sinus rhythm, in the setting of a narrow QRS, the first determination is whether it is regular or irregular. A regular rhythm is not always sinus rhythm. It can be driven by an ectopic atrial focus or by a reentrant tachyarrhythmia (one of the many SVTs). Irregular rhythms are characterized by variable intervals between QRS complexes. Irregular rhythms can be further divided into regularly irregular and irregularly irregular. A regularly irregular rhythm is defined by a predictable pattern in QRS intervals. Examples of this are atrial or ventricular bigeminy or trigeminy caused by premature atrial contractions or premature ventricular contractions. An irregularly irregular rhythm shows no pattern in the intervals between QRS complexes. Examples of such a rhythm are atrial fibrillation and multifocal atrial tachycardia. The next step in determining the rhythm is to define the P wave.

Step 4: The P Wave

The P wave represents atrial depolarization. Identifying the P wave can sometimes be challenging. The sinus P-wave morphology is positive in the inferior leads as described above. If a P wave is seen in front of the QRS complex, but it is negative in the inferior leads, it is likely coming from a different atrial focus. If a P wave cannot be seen, it is usually buried inside the QRS or the T wave. Such is the case in AV nodal reentry tachycardia or a junctional tachycardia. If a P wave is seen closer to the preceding QRS rather than the following QRS, a reentrant atrioventricular tachycardia should be suspected or an atrial rhythm with a long first-degree AV block. The width, shape, and amplitude of the P waves can inform about atrial enlargement. Left atrial enlargement (LAE) is likely present when a P wave's length is greater than 120 milliseconds in lead II. A notched P wave forming an "M"-like shape is frequently seen. The clearest example of this is mitral stenosis, but LAE is most often seen with longstanding hypertension. Right atrial enlargement is defined by a P wave's height of ≥2.5 mm in lead II. Right atrial enlargement is most often seen in patients with lung disease. When the P waves have ≥3 different morphologies, a wandering atrial pacemaker of a multifocal atrial tachycardia should be suspected.

Step 5: What Is the QRS Axis?

The axis that is usually referred to on the ECG is the axis of the QRS complex in the frontal plane. The axis correlates with the vector of the electrical impulse as it proceeds from the AV node through ventricular depolarization/contraction.

- *Normal QRS axis:* The direction of the vector described above results in a positive deflection in both the P wave and the QRS in leads I, II, and aVF. The most positive lead is lead II, which is closest in axis to the vector of a normal conduction system. Lead aVR is generally negative, because the vector is almost exactly the opposite of lead II. A normal QRS axis is typically between −30° and 90°.
- *Right-axis deviation:* Right QRS axis deviation occurs when lead I has a negative QRS deflection. Lead aVF and lead II generally remain positive. This occurs when the direction of depolarization is toward the right and the axis is ≥90°. Severe right-axis deviation is noted when leads I and II are also negative, and lead aVF is positive. Right-axis deviation is often seen in right ventricular hypertrophy, acute pulmonary embolus, chronic lung disease, or left posterior hemiblock.
- *Left-axis deviation (LAD):* Left QRS axis deviation is defined by a QRS axis ≤ −30°. Lead I is positive, and leads II and aVF are negative. LAD is generally

inconsequential. It can be seen in patients with hypertension, an old inferior myocardial infarction (MI), or a left anterior hemiblock.

Step 6: The QRS Complex

- *QRS duration*: The QRS complex measures the time of ventricular depolarization. The normal QRS duration is 70 to 100 milliseconds. A QRS duration of 100 to 120 milliseconds is described as an intraventricular conduction delay. A QRS ≥120 milliseconds defines a bundle branch block (right or left). Bundle branch blocks typically indicate conduction disease in the His-Purkinje system, below the AV node. They make the patient more likely to develop bradyarrhythmias, although many patients never do so. When the QRS complex is wide and the rate is tachycardic, the possibility of ventricular tachycardia needs to be ruled out.
- *QRS voltage:* In the setting of hypertension, the QRS voltage can increase because of LVH. This can also happen in patients with aortic stenosis. Several criteria for LVH have been described in the literature. At best, they are 50% to 60% sensitive and have been largely replaced by echocardiography.
- *QRS morphology:* In general, the QRS should start in most leads with a positive deflection. An initial negative deflection is named a Q wave. Normal Q waves are typically present in V5 and V6, as the normal initial septal depolarization, and in lead III, as a small isolated Q wave due to a normal QRS vector. Any Q wave in 2 contiguous leads lasting at least 0.04 seconds or one-third the amplitude of the QRS complex represents an old infarct.

Step 7: The Intervals

The portions of the ECG that are not P waves or QRS complexes are named intervals, as follows:

- *The PR interval* is measured from the beginning of the P wave, to the beginning of the QRS complex. The PR interval measures the time from the beginning of atrial depolarization to the end of atrial repolarization. A normal PR interval is 120 to 200 milliseconds. A short PR interval is seen in patients with Wolff-Parkinson-White syndrome or in normal young patients with rapid AV node conduction. A long PR interval is often seen in elderly patients with large atria or with slowed conduction across the atrial tissue.
- *QT interval:* The QT interval is measured from the beginning of the QRS complex to the end of the T wave. It represents ventricular depolarization and ventricular repolarization. It is one of the most difficult intervals to measure by a computerized algorithm. The QT interval varies with HR and is corrected for it (QTc). The QTc is calculated by dividing the measured QT in milliseconds by the square root of the R-R interval. An abnormal QTc is ≥480 milliseconds in men and ≥470 milliseconds in women. A prolonged QTc is associated with an increased risk of potentially fatal ventricular tachyarrhythmias, specifically, polymorphic ventricular tachycardia, known as Torsades de pointes. A prolonged QTc can be congenital or acquired. Many drugs and electrolyte abnormalities such as hyperkalemia can cause QTc prolongation.
- *TP interval:* The TP interval, the interval from the end of ventricular repolarization until the following atrial depolarization, is the most electrically silent portion of the ECG. As such, the TP interval is considered the true electrical baseline and should be used to assess ST segment elevation and depressions discussed later.

Step 8: Ischemic Evaluation

The final step in evaluating an ECG is to look for acute ischemic changes. In order to be significant, the ST segment changes or T-wave inversions have to be present in 2 concordant/contiguous leads representing a certain coronary territory. The coronary territories are defined as follows: (1) inferior: leads II, III, aVF; (2) lateral: leads I, aVL, V5, V6; (3) anterior: V1-V4.

- *ST segment elevation:* An elevation of at least 1 mm seen in 2 contiguous/concordant leads suggests an acute myocardial injury in the corresponding territory. Patients with chest pain and ST elevation are typically in the midst of an acute MI and should be referred immediately to the ED.
- *ST segment depression:* A depression of at least 1 mm seen in contiguous/concordant leads suggests either myocardial injury or myocardial ischemia. Patients with ST segment depressions may have either an acute MI or unstable angina. They too should be referred to the ED.
- *T-wave inversions:* Typically T waves should be positive where the QRS is positive and negative where the QRS is negative. When the T waves are inverted in contiguous/concordant leads, they can indicate either an old infarction or acute ischemia. To differentiate between the two, an old ECG is usually needed. Another cause for T-wave inversions is LVH with repolarization changes. In such cases, the T-wave morphology is typically asymmetrical, as opposed to ischemic T-wave changes, which are usually symmetric.

SUMMARY

An ECG is a simple test that can give the primary care physician important information on patients with risk factors and/or symptoms of CVD. The indications for an ECG in asymptomatic patients are few, because the likelihood of finding significant abnormalities is low. It is the primary care physician's responsibility to be proficient in the interpretation of an ECG because computerized algorithms, although improved, can give erroneous information. Approaching ECG interpretation in a stepwise, systematic manner is important to make sure ECG findings are not missed.

REFERENCES

1. Schneider JF, Thomas HE, Kreger BE, et al. Newly acquired right bundle-branch block: the Framingham study. Ann Intern Med 1980;92:37–44.
2. Schneider JF, Thomas HE, Sorlie P, et al. Comparative features of newly acquired left and right bundle branch block in the general population: the Framingham study. Am J Cardiol 1981;47:931–40.
3. Ashley EA, Raxwal VK, Froelicher VF. The prevalence and prognostic significance of electrocardiographic abnormalities. Curr Probl Cardiol 2000;25:1–72.
4. US Preventive Services Task Force recommendation statement. Screening for cardiovascular disease risk with electrocardiography. JAMA 2018;319:2308–14.
5. US Preventive Services Task Force Recommendation Statement. Screening for atrial fibrillation with electrocardiography. JAMA 2018;320(5):478–84.
6. Malhotra A, Dhutia H, Finocchiaro G, et al. Outcomes of cardiac screening in adolescent soccer players. N Engl J Med 2018;379:524–34.
7. Fleisher LA, Fleischmann KE, Auerbach AD, et al. 2014 ACC/AHA guideline on perioperative cardiovascular evaluation and management of patients undergoing noncardiac surgery a report of the American College of Cardiology/American

Heart Association Task Force on practice guidelines. Circulation 2014;130: e278–333.

8. Kristensen SD, Knuuti J. New ESC/ESA guidelines on non-cardiac surgery: cardiovascular assessment and management. Eur Heart J 2014;35:2344–5.

9. Duceppe E, Parlow J, MacDonald P, et al. Canadian Cardiovascular Society guidelines on perioperative cardiac risk assessment and management for patients who undergo noncardiac surgery. Can J Cardiol 2017;33:17–32.

10. De Hert S, Staender S, Fritsch G, et al. Pre-operative evaluation of adults undergoing elective noncardiac surgery: updated guideline from the European Society of Anaesthesiology. Eur J Anaesthesiol 2018;35:407–65.

11. Sgarbossa EB, Pinski SL, Barbagelata A, et al. Electrocardiographic diagnosis of evolving acute myocardial infarction in the presence of left bundle-branch block. N Engl J Med 1996;334:481–7.

12. Richard L, Page MD, José A, et al. 2015 ACC/AHA/HRS guideline for the management of adult patients with supraventricular tachycardia. J Am Coll Cardiol 2016;67:1575–623.

13. Guglin ME, Thatai D. Common errors in computer electrocardiogram interpretation. Int J Cardiol 2006;106:232–7.

14. Hwan Bae M, Hoon Lee J, Heon Yang D, et al. Erroneous computer ECG interpretation of atrial fibrillation and its clinical consequences. Clin Cardiol 2012;35: 348–53.

15. Jonathan S, Steinberg MD, Niraj Varma MD, et al. 2017 ISHNE-HRS expert consensus statement on ambulatory ECG and external cardiac monitoring. Heart Rhythm 2017;14:e55–96.

16. Salerno SM, Alguire PC, Waxman HS. Competency in interpretation of 12-lead electrocardiograms: a summary and appraisal of published evidence. Ann Intern Med 2003;138:751–60.

17. Antiperovitch P, Zareba W, Steinberg JS, et al. Proposed in-training electrocardiogram interpretation competencies for undergraduate and postgraduate trainees. J Hosp Med 2017;13:185–93.

18. Kadish AH, Buxton AE, Kennedy HL, et al. ACC/AHA clinical competence statement on ECGs and ambulatory ECGs: a report of the ACC/AHA/ACP–ASIM task force on clinical competence. Circulation 2001;104:3169–78.

19. Dubin D. Rapid interpretation of EKG's. 6th edition. Fort Myers(FL): 2000.

20. Wagner GS, Strauss DG. Marriott's practical electrocardiography. 12th edition. Philadelphia: Wolters Kluwer|Lippincott Williams & Wilkins; 2014. p. 532.

Palpitation
Extended Electrocardiogram Monitoring: Which Tests to Use and When

Kara J. Quan, MD, FHRS*

KEYWORDS

- Palpitation • Extended monitoring • Holter • Event • Implantable loop recorder

KEY POINTS

- It is important to tailor evaluation based on patient's symptoms.
- Twenty-four-hour Holter monitoring is useful if symptoms occur daily.
- If symptoms are less frequent, an external continuous monitor (2 week to 30 days) may be helpful.
- If symptoms occur monthly or less frequently, cardiology referral for an implantable loop recorder is optimal.

INTRODUCTION

Palpitation is a very common symptom for which patients present to their primary care physician, cardiologist, or the emergency room. It is often accompanied by other symptoms that can portend a more malignant prognosis, such as lightheadedness, near syncope, or syncope. Although most of the time palpitation are benign, they may be very debilitating to the patient. In terms of quality of life, it is often important to document what the symptoms are from to reassure the patient. However, it may be difficult to confirm a diagnosis in patients with infrequent symptoms. When this symptom remains unexplained after a routine history, physical examination, and 12-lead electrocardiogram (ECG), other forms of monitoring may be indicated. A diagnostic plan with external monitoring tools such as a 24-hour Holter monitor, an extended continuous loop external monitor, or an implantable loop recorder may be used. Up until the late 1990s, the technology was limited and there were few data and few options for noninvasive rhythm monitoring.[1] However, over the last decade the technology used for external monitoring has improved significantly. In fact, there are now several kinds of devices, and which device is better suited for individual

Disclosure Statement: I have no disclosures.
Case Western Reserve University, Cleveland, OH, USA
* 125 East Broad Street, Suite 305, Elyria, OH 44035.
E-mail address: kquan@nohc.com

Med Clin N Am 103 (2019) 785–791
https://doi.org/10.1016/j.mcna.2019.05.005
0025-7125/19/© 2019 Elsevier Inc. All rights reserved.

patients has become more difficult to ascertain. Recent guidelines published by the Heart Rhythm Society are helpful in this regard.[2] In this article, the author reviews the data for the role of 24-hour monitoring, continuous loop external monitoring, and implantable loop recorder in the workup of patients with palpitation.

Palpitation may result from different types of arrhythmias, such as premature atrial or ventricular contractions, sinus nodal dysfunction, advanced atrioventricular block, and sustained or nonsustained supraventricular or ventricular tachycardia. Often, such palpitations are associated with dizziness, near syncope, or syncope. A thorough history and physical examination are important. Because the examination often occurs when the patient is asymptomatic, the examination is mostly directed at determining the presence of any underlying cardiac disease. If there are signs or symptoms of cardiac disease on history or examination, such as murmurs or evidence of volume overload, an echocardiogram is indicated. However, the following discussion applies for the most part to patients who have a normal cardiac examination.

ELECTROCARDIOGRAM EVALUATION

A baseline 12-lead ECG is important in all patients with symptoms of palpitation. The ECG offers important information in the evaluation for underlying cardiac abnormalities. One can detect prior myocardial infarction, a short PR interval and delta wave indicative of Wolff–Parkinson–White syndrome, a long QT interval, left ventricular hypertrophy, right ventricular hypertrophy, atrial enlargement, or atrioventricular block. In the presence of an abnormal ECG, further diagnostic testing is indicated to rule out significant structural heart disease. Echocardiography, stress testing, and referral to a cardiologist or electrophysiologist are often indicated.

TWENTY-FOUR HOUR HOLTER MONITORING

In the past 24-hour Holter monitoring was the cornerstone of the diagnostic tools available to the clinician for the diagnosis of palpitation. Today, it is indicated mostly in patients whose symptoms clearly occur within the period of monitoring. For example, in patients whose palpitation occur daily or several times daily, a 24-hour monitor will be helpful. This simple device is worn continuously for 24 hours. The patient keeps a log of any symptoms that occur during testing. The monitor is then returned to a technician, scanned, analyzed, and then given to a physician for a final report. Holter monitors tend to be expensive monitoring devices and are maintained by outpatient clinics or hospitals. The results of a 24-hour Holter monitor are diagnostic only in 10% to 15% of patients with palpitation. If palpitations correlate with sinus rhythm on the recorder, the patient can be reassured. In patients who experience syncope, the diagnosis can be made by Holter monitor only 5% to 10% of the time. Longer term monitors are much more effective for this purpose because, by nature, syncope typically occurs less than once a day. With Holter monitoring, symptomatic premature atrial complexes or symptomatic premature ventricular complexes are often detected, and in such cases, especially if the patient has a structurally normal heart, the patient can be reassured. If nonsustained or sustained ventricular or supraventricular arrhythmias are detected, then treatment of the arrhythmia and referral to a cardiologist may be appropriate. Another area where 24-hour Holter monitors are still useful is in patients with palpitation and persistent or permanent atrial fibrillation. In such patients, it is often difficult to assess the ventricular rate control by ECG alone. A 24-hour Holter monitor is very helpful in determining whether the ventricular response is well-controlled during daily activities in patients who complain of shortness of breath or palpitations.[3]

EXTERNAL CARDIAC EVENT MONITORS

For the most part, in the diagnosis and management of palpitation, 24-hour Holter monitors have been replaced by longer term external event monitors. These devices are fitted in the hospital or at home. They are worn between 7 and 30 days, depending on patients' preference. They transmit data via cell phone or cellular networks to a centralized station. Some monitors are self-contained monitors that are sent back to a centralized station for downloading. The patient wears a continuous loop event monitor at all times for up to a month. These monitors save data only for the previous and subsequent few minutes after the patient manually activates the monitor. Most devices now have an autotriggered mode, where the device automatically records, stores, and transmits an arrhythmia if it meets the criteria for a rapid rate or a very slow rate. Another type of external cardiac event monitor is not worn continuously, but is carried by the patient, and transmissions are sent when the patient has symptoms. With the latter type of intermittent monitoring, a few minutes of data may be saved, but the onset of the arrhythmia may be missed. Finally, a newer type of recorder, named mobile cardiac telemetry, records all data for up to 30 days. The data from this type of monitor are sent to a centralized location where technicians review the telemetry on a real-time basis and inform the patient (and the physician) in real time if an arrhythmia is detected. This type of device is similar to a patient being monitored as an in-patient on a telemetry floor. A very good description of first- and second-generation external ambulatory event monitors can be found in the 2017 International Society for Holter and NonInvasive Electrocardiography Expert Consensus statement on Ambulatory ECG and External Cardiac Telemetry.[2]

SELECTION OF AMBULATORY MONITORING DEVICES

Studies have compared the diagnostic yield of Holter monitoring and external cardiac monitors. Twenty-four-hour Holter monitoring was diagnostic in 10% to 15% of patients with palpitation, whereas event monitoring had a diagnostic yield of 66% to 83%. In retrospective and prospective trials, 83% to 87% of patients had diagnostic transmissions within 2 weeks of using an event monitor.[4,5] If a patient has daily episodes of palpitation, then a 24-hour Holter monitor is recommended for evaluation. Otherwise, the event monitor is much more likely to yield a diagnosis. It should be noted that a 48-hour Holter has not been shown to be superior to a 24-hour recording.[6]

Although there are clear advantages in monitoring for prolonged periods of time, one drawback is patient compliance. Scherr and colleagues[7] reported that "leadless" pocket sized, portable, intermittent cardiac event monitors showed a patient compliance of 100% compared with a compliance of 78% in patients wearing a continuous loop recorder for 30 days. There was no difference in the frequency of symptomatic episodes or the number of recorded arrhythmias. In addition, 2 weeks of monitoring with a leadless device had a much higher yield of arrhythmias than a 24-hour Holter monitor.[8] Additionally, asymptomatic arrhythmias may be discovered during extended event monitoring. Locati and colleagues[9] determined that 13% of patients had clinically significant, asymptomatic arrhythmias that were automatically detected by the autotrigger feature of the device. The patients included in their study had palpitation, presyncope, or unexplained syncope. Therefore, external event recorders with automatically triggered events are much more helpful than 24-hour Holter monitors in the diagnosis tachyarrhythmias or bradyarrhythmias in patients with syncope or infrequent palpitation. Furthermore, external event monitoring is more cost effective than Holter monitoring. Zimetbaum and colleagues[10,11] determined that continuous loop recorders had a diagnostic yield of 1.04 diagnoses per patient in week 1; 0.15

diagnoses per patient in week 2, and 0.01 diagnoses per patient in week 3 and beyond. Part of that is driven by the fact that patients are less likely to wear the monitor as time goes by. As a result, over time, the cost effectiveness ratio increased from $98 per new diagnosis in week 1 to $576 per new diagnosis in week 2 to $5832 per new diagnosis in week 3. Therefore, most experts recommend a period of external monitoring of between 2 and 4 weeks, with the 2-week period of monitoring being the most cost effective.

The technology of external cardiac event recorders has now evolved to the ability to record and monitor telemetry in real time. With MCT monitors, patients wear a monitor that wirelessly transmits continuous telemetry recordings to a centralized location staffed by trained technicians 24 hours a day. With such devices patients are monitored as if they were in the hospital. If a life-threatening bradyarrhythmia or tachyarrhythmia is recorded, the technician can call the patient immediately and advise them to go to the emergency department or activate a 911 dispatch directly. The MCT recorders are particularly useful to detect the burden of atrial fibrillation in patients who have had pulmonary vein isolation and for patients at risk for life-threatening arrhythmias such as after bypass surgery or after transcutaneous aortic valve replacement procedures.

In summary, data support the use of 2 to 4 weeks of external cardiac event recorders over 24-hour Holter monitoring in the workup of patients with palpitation, unless the patient has daily symptoms. If symptoms persist, are not well-tolerated, or cannot be diagnosed accurately, a referral to an electrophysiologist may be reasonable to consider the implantation of an internal loop recorder.

IMPLANTABLE LOOP RECORDERS

When a diagnosis cannot be made with an external loop recorder because the symptoms of palpitation, near syncope, or syncope are too infrequent, or because the patient cannot tolerate wearing the monitor, a new device, which is implantable in the subcutaneous tissue, is now available. The implantable loop recorder is a small device, about the size of a flattened ballpoint pen cap, that is implanted subcutaneously in the left precordial area, just left of the sternum in the fourth to fifth intercostal space. The procedure is done as an outpatient, takes 15 to 30 minutes, and carries an extremely low risk burden. The device is a self-contained system that has 2 electrodes 2 inches apart to detect electrical activity continuously. The nonrechargeable battery has a life expectancy of about 3 years on average and can provide continuous monitoring for even longer than that. The patient is provided with a monitoring box that sends information via the Internet to a centralized station. The patient's device clinic then downloads the information from the Internet at scheduled dates, typically once a month. In addition, any event that is recorded as abnormal by the device, based on programmed parameters, is transmitted automatically to the clinic as an alert. Further, when the patients are symptomatic, they can activate the recorder and transmit to the clinic. In that way, symptoms can be correlated with the rhythm to rule out or rule in a tachyarrhythmia or bradyarrhythmia. There had been no data for the usefulness of an implantable loop recorder in the diagnosis of palpitation of unknown cause, until the recent publication by Giada and colleagues[12] of the Recurrent Unexplained Palpitations (RUP) Study. These investigators compared the diagnostic yield and cost of an implantable loop recorder with a conventional strategy in patients with unexplained palpitation. After an initial evaluation by history, physical examination, and ECG, 50 patients were randomized in a multicenter prospective study to a conventional diagnostic strategy versus an implantable loop recorder. The conventional

Table 1
Baseline clinical characteristics

Baseline Characteristics	Conventional (n = 24)	Implantable Loop (n = 26)
Age, years, mean ± SD	43 ± 17	51 ± 18
Female, %	79	54
Palpitation episodes in last year, median	6	8
Length of episodes, minutes, median	40	51
Duration of symptoms, months, median	30	44
LVEF, %, mean ± SD	63 ± 6	60 ± 7
Structural heart disease, n (%)	6 (25)	11 (42)
Hypertension	5	7
Ischemic heart disease	1	—
Valvular heart disease	—	3
Dilated cardiomyopathy	—	1

Abbreviations: LVEF, left ventricular ejection fraction; SD, standard deviation.

diagnostic strategy included a 24-hour Holter monitor followed by an external cardiac event monitor, and then an electrophysiologic study.

In the RUP study, patients had a negative initial evaluation including history, physical examination, and ECG. Patients were randomized to either conventional strategy (24-hour Holter monitoring, 4-week ambulatory ECG monitoring with an external cardiac event monitor, and an electrophysiologic study) or to an implantable loop recorder with a 1-year monitoring period. Hospital costs of the 2 strategies were compared. There were no differences in baseline clinical characteristics between groups (**Table 1**). A diagnosis for the etiology of palpitation was found in 60% patients. Of these patients, 73% had a significant arrhythmia diagnoses (**Table 2**).

The primary end point of establishing the cause of palpitation was achieved in 21% of patients in the conventional strategy group. The mean time to diagnosis was 36 ± 26 days. The 24-hour Holter monitors were negative in all patients. With

Table 2
Diagnostic outcome

	Conventional (n = 24)	Implantable Loop (n = 26)
Diagnosis made, n (%)	5 (21)	19 (73)
Supraventricular tachycardia	4	6
Atrial fibrillation/flutter	1	6
Sinus tachycardia	0	4
Sinus bradycardia	0	2
Paroxysmal atrioventricular block	0	1
No diagnosis, n (%)	19 (79)	7 (27)
No palpitation	16	6
Patient error with device	5	1
Device malfunction	1	0
Negative electrophysiologic study	19	—

Abbreviation: SD, standard deviation.

Box 1
Diagnoses in the conventional strategies and implantable loop recorder groups

Conventional strategies (n = 24)
  Diagnosis n = 5 (21%)
  No diagnosis n = 19 (79%)

Crossover to implantable loop recorder (n = 9)
  Diagnosis n = 6 (67%)
  No diagnosis n = 3 (33%)

Implantable loop recorder (n = 26)
  Diagnosis n = 19 (73%)
  No diagnosis n = 7 (27%)

30-day cardiac event monitoring, 1 patient was found to have atrial fibrillation, and 1 patient had supraventricular tachycardia. With electrophysiological testing, 3 patients had inducible supraventricular tachycardia. Nondiagnostic testing occurred in 79% patients in the conventional group (n = 19). Of those, 9 patients crossed over to the implantable loop recorder arm. Subsequently, a diagnosis was obtained in 67% of them with a mean time to diagnosis of 316 ± 226 days. Supraventricular tachycardia, sinus tachycardia, or paroxysmal atrioventricular block were the diagnoses (**Box 1**). In the implantable loop recorder group, a diagnosis was obtained in 73% of patients. The mean time to diagnosis was 279 ± 228 days. The diagnoses were supraventricular tachycardia, atrial fibrillation, atrial flutter, sinus tachycardia, sinus bradycardia, and paroxysmal atrioventricular block.

With regard to cost, the mean cost per patient was higher in the implantable loop recorder group compared with the conventional strategy group. However, the mean cost per diagnosis was significantly lower in the implantable loop recorder group. Overall, it was more cost effective to implant a loop recorder, which was much more likely to obtain a firm diagnosis in patients with unexplained palpitation (**Table 3**).

In follow-up, patients who were diagnosed with an arrhythmia as the etiology of the palpitation had either elimination or reduction of symptoms after ablation, antiarrhythmic medications, or pacemaker implantation. Patients with a nonarrhythmic etiology of palpitation were treated with anxiolytic medications. Overall, patients with infrequent symptoms of palpitation and no significant structural heart disease were more likely to have a diagnosis with an implantable loop recorder rather than conventional strategy.

Implantable loop recorders have also been shown to be beneficial in patients with unexplained recurrent syncope, when the episodes are fairly far apart.[13] Moreover,

---

Table 3
Cost of testing

	Conventional (n = 24)	Implantable Loop (n = 26)	P value
Cost per patient			
Cost of testing, mean ± SD	$1410 ± 1389	$2233 ± 265	.001
Cost per diagnosis			
Cost of testing, mean ± SD	$6768 ± 6672	$3056 ± 363	.012

Abbreviation: SD, standard deviation.

they have a role in detecting silent atrial tachyarrhythmias, specifically asymptomatic atrial fibrillation or atrial flutter in patients with unexplained (cryptogenic) strokes.[14]

SUMMARY

Noninvasive evaluation of palpitation should be tailored to the patient's symptoms. Depending on the frequency of symptoms, an external monitor can be used. If there are daily symptoms, a 24-hour Holter monitor is useful. If there are infrequent symptoms, a 2 to 4 week cardiac event monitor is more likely to yield a diagnosis than a 24-hour Holter monitor. If the symptoms are even less frequent, then an implantable loop recorder and referral to cardiology or electrophysiology is the optimal option.

REFERENCES

1. Weber BE, Kapoor WH. Evaluations and outcomes of patients with palpitations. Am J Med 1999;338:1369–73.
2. Steinberg JS, Varma N, Cygankiewicz I, et al. 2017 ISHNE-HRS expert consensus statement on ambulatory ECG and external cardiac monitoring/telemetry. Heart Rhythm 2017;14:e55–96.
3. VanGelder IC, Rienstra M, Crijns HJ, et al. Rate control in atrial fibrillation. Lancet 2016;388:818–28.
4. Zimetbaum PJ, Josephson ME. Evolving role of ambulatory monitoring in general clinical practice. Ann Intern Med 1999;130:848–67.
5. Kohno R, Abe H, Benditt DG. Ambulatory electrocardiogram monitoring devices for evaluating transient loss of consciousness or other related symptoms. J Arrhythm 2017;33:583–9.
6. Kennedy HL, Chandra V, Sayther KL, et al. Effectiveness of increasing hours of continuous ambulatory electrocardiography in detecting maximal ventricular ectopy: continuous 48 hour study of patients with coronary heart disease and normal subjects. Am J Cardiol 1978;42:925–30.
7. Scherr D, Dalal D, Henrikson CA, et al. Prospective comparison of diagnostic utility of standard event monitor versus a leadless portable ECG monitor in the evaluation of patients with palpitations. J Interv Card Electrophysiol 2008;22:39–44.
8. Barrett PM, Komatireddy R, Haaser S, et al. Comparison of 24-hour Holter monitoring with 14-day novel adhesive patch electrocardiographic monitoring. Am J Med 2017;127:95.e11-7.
9. Locati ET, Vecchi AM, Vargiu S, et al. Role of extended loop recorders for diagnosis of unexplained syncope, pre-syncope, and sustained palpitations. Europace 2014;16:914–22.
10. Zimetbaum PJ, Kim KY, Josephson ME, et al. Diagnostic yield and optimal duration of continuous loop event monitoring for diagnosis of palpitations. A cost effectiveness analysis. Ann Intern Med 1998;128:890–5.
11. Tsang JP, Mohan S. Benefits of monitoring patients with mobile cardiac telemetry (MCT) compared with the event or Holter monitors. Med Devices (Auckl) 2014;7:1–5.
12. Giada F, Gulizia M, Francese M, et al. Recurrent unexplained palpitations study. J Am Coll Cardiol 2007;49(19):1951–6.
13. Tanno K. Use of implantable and external loop recorders in syncope with unknown causes. J Arrhythm 2017;33:579–82.
14. Sanna T, Diener HC, Passman RS, et al. Cryptogenic stroke and underlying atrial fibrillation; the CRYSTAL AF Investigators. N Engl J Med 2014;370(26):2478–86.

When Is Syncope Arrhythmic?

Evan Martow, BMSc, MDCM[a], Roopinder Sandhu, MD, MPH[b],*

KEYWORDS

- Arrhythmia • Syncope • Bradyarrhythmia • Tachyarrhythmia • Cardiac monitoring

KEY POINTS

- Syncope is a symptom that presents with an abrupt, transient, and complete loss of consciousness associated with inability to maintain postural tone, with rapid and spontaneous recovery.
- Arrhythmic syncope (a subcategory of cardiac syncope) can be a result of bradyarrhythmia (due to sinus node dysfunction and/or atrioventricular node or distal conduction system disease) or tachyarrhythmia (due to ventricular tachycardia or supraventricular tachycardia).
- Initial evaluation should include a history, physical examination, and 12-lead electrocardiogram (ECG). If the cause remains unclear, a high clinical suspicion for arrhythmic cause will guide further testing and cardiac monitoring.
- The goal of cardiac monitoring is to obtain symptom–rhythm correlation. The choice of cardiac monitoring device should be guided by the frequency of symptoms and the likelihood that the patient may be incapacitated and, therefore, cannot voluntarily trigger the ECG recording device.
- Referral to a heart rhythm specialist should be considered if high-risk features are present on initial evaluation to expedite treatment, when the significance of findings is uncertain, or when there is high suspicion of an arrhythmic cause requiring further management.

DEFINITION

Syncope is defined as an

- Abrupt, transient, complete loss of consciousness
- Associated with inability to maintain postural tone
- With rapid and spontaneous recovery
- With the absence of clinical features of alternative causes, such as seizure, head trauma, psychogenic pseudosyncope.[1]

The authors have nothing to disclose.
[a] Division of Cardiology, University of Alberta, University of Alberta Hospital, Walter Mackenzie Health Sciences Centre, 8440 112 Street, Edmonton, Alberta T6G 2B7, Canada; [b] Division of Cardiology, University of Alberta, Walter Mackenzie Health Sciences Centre, 8440 112 Street, Edmonton, Alberta T6G 2B7, Canada
* Corresponding author.
E-mail address: rsandhu2@ualberta.ca

Presyncope symptoms, including extreme lightheadedness; visual sensations, such as tunnel vision; and varying degrees of altered level of consciousness, may occur before a syncopal event or resolve without syncope.[1]

CAUSES OF SYNCOPE

Syncope causes can be categorized as noncardiac or cardiac (**Fig. 1**). Arrhythmia is a common cause of cardiac syncope and can be further subdivided into bradyarrhythmias and tachyarrhythmias.

Bradyarrhythmias are caused by

- Sinus node dysfunction (historically dubbed sick sinus syndrome), which includes inappropriate sinus bradycardia[a], sinus pause[b], atrial arrest,[c] sinoatrial exit block[d], and tachy-brady syndrome[e]
- Atrioventricular (AV) node or conduction system dysfunction (prolonged PR interval, second-degree type I and II AV block, third-degree AV block).[2]

Bradyarrhythmias result in syncope due to inadequate cerebral perfusion from slow rates or missed beats.

Tachyarrhythmias can be mediated by tissues above the level of the ventricle (supraventricular) or within the ventricle itself. Supraventricular tachycardia (SVT) describes tachycardia (atrial and/or ventricular rates >100 beats per minute) driven by tissue from the His bundle or above.[3] Examples include AV reentrant tachycardia (AVRT), AV nodal reentrant tachycardia (AVNRT), atrial tachycardia (AT), atrial flutter, and atrial fibrillation. Ventricular tachycardia (VT) can occur in monomorphic and/or polymorphic forms.[4] Tachyarrhythmias result in syncope due to inadequate cardiac filling with corresponding poor cardiac output and cerebral perfusion.

Malfunctions in cardiac implanted devices can also result in syncope. If a pacemaker malfunctions, the underlying bradyarrhythmia may cause syncope. Additionally, cardiac devices can be implicated in pacemaker-mediated tachycardias, which can cause syncope.[5]

Arrhythmic Syncope: Epidemiology and Diagnosis

Syncope is a common presentation to emergency departments, accounting for an estimated 1% to 6% of all visits annually. A high proportion of these patients are hospitalized, ranging from 13% to 86%.[6-8] The most common causes of syncope are reflex syncope (~20%), followed by cardiac syncope (~10%) and orthostatic syncope (~10%).[1] Arrhythmic syncope represents a significant proportion of cardiac syncope cases. However, varying definitions, inclusion or exclusion criteria, and diagnostic approaches have led to wide variation in the reported proportions of syncope attributed to arrhythmia.[9-12]

Arrhythmic syncope can be caused by either bradyarrhythmia or tachyarrhythmia. The objective of monitoring for arrhythmic syncope is achieving symptom–rhythm correlation: if the patient reports symptoms coinciding with rhythm abnormalities

---

[a] Rate less than 50 beats per minute with symptoms.

[b] Less than 3-second delay between depolarization.

[c] Absence of atrial depolarization.

[d] Inability of sinus node to depolarize atrium.

[e] Presence of periods of sinus node dysfunction and abnormal tachycardia (eg, atrial fibrillation) potentially with pauses at termination of tachycardia.

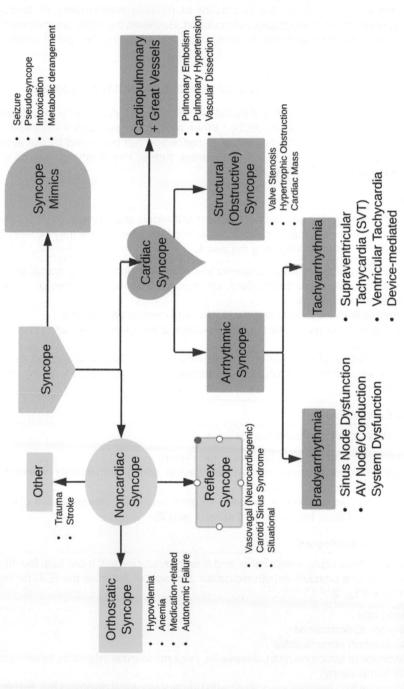

Fig. 1. Causes of syncope. AV, atrioventricular.

on a cardiac monitor, this will clinch the diagnosis.[13] Additionally, if a patient has a symptomatic event while on a cardiac monitor that shows no significant arrhythmia, this typically excludes a rhythm disorder as the cause of their symptoms. Of course, the possibility of multiple mechanisms of syncope should be considered, in the appropriate context. However, capturing an episode during a patient's initial presentation is uncommon, necessitating the use of additional tools.

IDENTIFYING AN ARRHYTHMIC CAUSE OF SYNCOPE ON INITIAL EVALUATION

Initial evaluation for syncope should include a thorough history, physical examination, and a 12-lead electrocardiogram (ECG).[1] When a cause for syncope is identified, the underlying mechanism can be treated, and disposition can be guided by risk stratification. If the cause for syncope is not apparent, further investigations may be warranted to identify the cause (**Fig. 2**).

History

A detailed history (gathered from both patient self-report and bystanders) is the most important aspect for evaluating the cause of syncope and key details may increase the suspicion for arrhythmia underlying the event:

- Situation in which syncope occurred (especially relationship to physical activity)
- Prodromal symptoms (palpitations, presyncope, nausea, diaphoresis)
- Postevent symptoms
- Comorbidities (especially cardiovascular and cardiac risk factors)
- Medications (focus on heart rate modulators, antihypertensives, and QT interval prolongers)
- Family history of syncope and/or premature (age <50 years) sudden cardiac death (including drowning, single-vehicle collisions, sudden infant death syndrome)

Physical Examination

A physical examination should include

- Vital signs, with focus on heart rate and rhythm
- Postural blood pressure and heart rate (laying, sitting, immediately on standing, and after 3 minutes of standing)
- Precordial examination for evidence of structural heart disease (valve disease, chamber dilation, heart failure) (**Tables 1** and **2**).

12-Lead Electrocardiogram

A 12-lead ECG is a rapid, inexpensive, and readily available test. It can help identify or provide clues to a possible arrhythmic cause of syncope. Examine the ECG for high-risk features (**Fig. 3**)[1,2,4,8,11,14,15]:

- Heart rate
- Rhythm abnormalities
- Conduction abnormalities
- Evidence of structural heart disease (ie, prior myocardial infarction, hypertrophic cardiomyopathy)
- Characteristic features associated with primary electrical disorders (eg, Brugada, long QT syndrome).

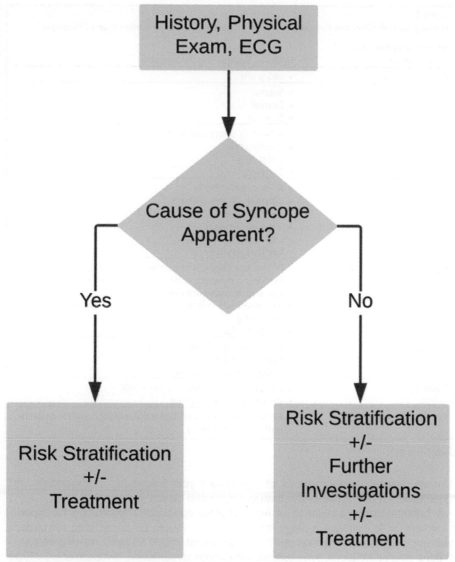

Fig. 2. Initial evaluation of syncope.

RISK STRATIFICATION AND DISPOSITION

Risk stratification is important to estimate prognosis, influence the decision for hospitalization, and establish the urgency of specialist involvement. To reduce unnecessary hospitalizations and reduce health care costs, numerous emergency department syncope risk tools[11,16–20] were developed to aid in physician decision-making. However, owing to important limitations (inconsistent definitions of syncope, outcomes, outcome time frames and predictors, small sample size, and limited external validation), these tools have not been widely adopted. Overall, these studies did demonstrate that an abnormal ECG, increasing age, and data suggesting structural heart

Table 1
History and physical examination features suggesting an arrhythmic cause of syncope

History and Physical Examination	Features Suggesting Arrhythmia
Age	• >65 y old
Context	• Supine • Seated • Exercise
Prodrome	• Absent or short prodrome • Palpitations • Chest pain • Dizziness
Comorbidities	• Known arrhythmia • Coronary artery disease • Heart failure • Valvular disease • Low ejection fraction • Cardiomyopathy
Family history	• Premature (age<50 y) sudden cardiac death (sudden, unexpected death from known cardiac cause or if cause unknown) • Single-vehicle collision • Drowning • Sudden infant death syndrome
Medications	• QT interval prolonging agents • Rate-control agents • Antiarrhythmic agents
Vital signs	• Abnormal heart rate (<50 or >100) • Abnormal heart rhythm
Precordial examination	• Evidence of structural heart disease (eg, dilated ventricle, pathologic murmur)

Data from Refs[1,10,14–16]

disease have a worse prognosis at 1-year to 2-year follow-up.[1,21] Importantly, risk tools have not performed better than unstructured clinical judgment.[22]

A hospital-based evaluation or heart rhythm specialist consultation to expedite treatment or to continue a diagnostic evaluation should be considered for patients with documented arrhythmias (sustained or symptomatic VT, second-degree type II or third-degree AV block, symptomatic sinus node dysfunction, symptomatic SVT, device malfunction) or when there is a high suspicion of an arrhythmia based on history, physical examination, and/or abnormal ECG.

ADDITIONAL INVESTIGATIONS

The use of additional investigations should be driven by the history, physical examination, and 12-lead resting ECG performed during the initial evaluation of syncope. A working hypothesis and differential diagnosis for an arrhythmic cause of syncope is imperative to determine the need and extent for further testing.

If structural heart disease is suspected, imaging with transthoracic echocardiography is useful, widely available, and low-risk.[23,24] Echocardiography can provide a clear cause of cardiac syncope; for example, by identifying significant valvular disease (ie, aortic stenosis). However, more often, it provides information regarding a potential

Table 2
Potential causes of arrhythmic syncope by age

Younger (<65 y)	Bradyarrhythmias • Conduction system dysfunction, including AV node and distal conduction disease (eg, due to sarcoidosis or Lyme disease) Tachyarrhythmias • SVT (AVNRT, AVRT, AT) • Atrial fibrillation • Long QT syndrome • Short QT syndrome • Arrhythmogenic right ventricular dysplasia • Catecholaminergic polymorphic VT • Idiopathic VT (eg, ventricular outflow tract VT) • Brugada syndrome
Older (>65 y)	Bradyarrhythmias • Sinus node dysfunction (sick sinus syndrome) • Conduction disease Tachyarrhythmias • Atrial fibrillation or flutter • AT • Acute ischemia VT (typically polymorphic) • Scar-mediated VT (monomorphic)

More common arrhythmias according to age but not representing a hard cutoff; arrhythmias in either category can present at any age.
Data from Refs.[17–23]

disease substrate (ie, hypertrophic cardiomyopathy, left ventricular [LV] dysfunction), which may have led to an arrhythmia.[25,26] For selected patients, when the echocardiography is inconclusive, advanced cardiac imaging (computed tomography or MRI) should be considered.[27,28] MRI is useful when there is suspicion for infiltrative disease, such as arrhythmogenic right ventricular cardiomyopathy (ARVC) or sarcoidosis. MRI is also helpful in detecting scar caused by prior myocarditis, or ischemic or nonischemic cardiomyopathy, any of which are a potential substrate for ventricular tachyarrhythmia.[29,30] Although exercise-induced syncope is uncommon, if a history is obtained of syncope during or immediately after exercise, then exercise stress testing should be performed and may unmask primary electrical disorders such as the long QT syndrome-1, catecholaminergic polymorphic VT (CPVT), or exercise-induced second-degree or third-degree AV block.[12,31]

The use of ambulatory cardiac monitoring should be based on a high suspicion for an arrhythmic cause. The type of monitor should take into consideration the frequency of syncope events, duration of monitoring, continuous versus intermittent recording, adequate prodrome, and sudden incapacitation. Symptom–rhythm correlation is the gold standard for the diagnosis of arrhythmic syncope. However, often, cardiac monitors detect asymptomatic arrhythmias, which may or may not be related to the presenting syncopal event. This presents a clinical dilemma for the health care provider. For these cases, an evaluation by a heart rhythm specialist can assist in interpretation and management.

The different types of cardiac monitors are summarized in **Table 3**. Although 24-hour Holter monitors are almost reflexively ordered during a syncope workup, the yield is very low (1%–2%). This is mainly because syncope recurrence does not typically occur during such a short monitoring period.[32–35] External loop recorders provide a higher yield than 24-hour Holter monitors because of a longer monitoring period and they have the additional advantages of recording both autotriggered

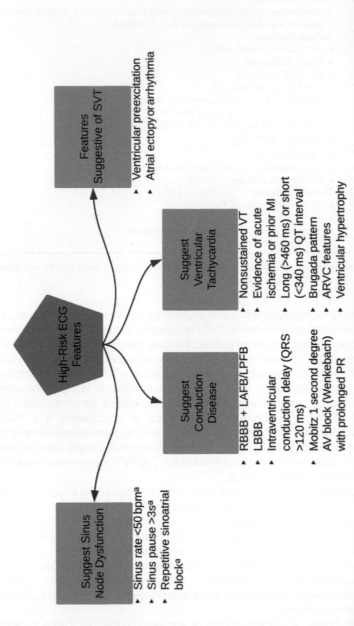

Fig. 3. High-risk ECG features. [a] In the absence of rate-lowering medications or physical training. ARVC, arrhythmogenic right ventricular cardiomyopathy; MI, myocardial infarction.

Table 3
Cardiac monitor descriptions

Cardiac Monitor	Monitor Description	Duration	Continuous or Intermittent	Patient Selection
Holter	Comprised of ECG electrode patches applied to chest, electrodes connected by wire leads to a battery-operated recording device	24–48 h	Continuous	Daily symptoms
External loop recorder	Comprised of ECG electrode patches applied to chest, electrodes connected by wire leads to a battery-operated recording device	2–6 wk	Continuous Autotriggered and patient-triggered	Weekly, spontaneous symptoms
External patch recorders	No leads or wires, adhesive to chest wall	2–14 d	Continuous	Weekly, spontaneous symptoms Alternative to external loop
Mobile cardiac outpatient telemetry	Comprising ECG electrode patches applied to chest, electrodes connected by wire leads Communication hub at home Transmission of ECG data through wireless network to a central monitoring station Real-time feedback	Up to 30 d	Continuous Autotriggered and patient-triggered	Weekly, spontaneous symptoms Real-time monitoring
Implantable cardiac monitor	Small, subcutaneously implanted device	≤3 y	Intermittent Autotriggered and patient-triggered	Recurrent, infrequent symptoms

(asymptomatic arrhythmias) and patient-triggered events (triggering can be activated before, during, or after symptoms).[36–39]

Newer technologies, including external patch recorders[40,41] and portable or wearable devices, are also available. These options provide only single-lead ECG recordings but are less cumbersome to the patient due to the absence of leads or wires. Further research is needed to better define the role of new technologies in the evaluation of arrhythmic syncope. Mobile cardiac outpatient telemetry also records autotriggered and patient-triggered events, as well as provides real-time arrhythmia monitoring and feedback to interpreting physicians.[42,43] This is unlike other noninvasive monitors for which rhythm interpretation occurs after the monitoring period is complete.

In patients with recurrent, infrequent syncope of suspected arrhythmic cause, an implantable cardiac monitor (implantable loop recorder) should be considered. Several randomized clinical trials and observational studies have demonstrated higher diagnostic yield compared with conventional testing.[44–49] The cost-effectiveness of an early implantable cardiac monitor strategy highly depends on the selected population, the pricing of devices, and the health care setting.[46,48,49]

The role of an invasive electrophysiology study (EPS) is limited to selected patients for whom there is a high suspicion of arrhythmic syncope, abnormal ECG, or structural heart disease. It should only be considered after noninvasive testing has been inconclusive and in consultation with a heart rhythm specialist.[50–52] EPS may also be considered in patients with cardiac sarcoidosis[53] or Brugada ECG pattern[54] and syncope of suspected arrhythmic cause.

MANAGEMENT OF ARRHYTHMIC SYNCOPE

When feasible, a heart rhythm specialist should be consulted for the management of arrhythmic syncope. General management approaches follow.

Bradyarrhythmias

In general, cardiac pacing therapy is indicated for intrinsic sinus node disease and AV conduction system disease associated with symptoms and documented by ECG.[1,22,55,56] When the correlation between symptoms and ECG is not established, cardiac pacing may still be reasonable in patients with unexplained syncope and trifascicular block, second-degree AV block, or long ($\geq$5 seconds) asymptomatic sinus pauses. In these situations, it is important to inform the patient that syncope may be caused by other mechanisms and recur, despite cardiac pacing therapy. Any drugs that may worsen or unmask bradycardia should be eliminated, when possible. In select cases, such as tachy-brady syndrome, cardiac ablation may be performed to control the atrial tachyarrhythmia.

Tachyarrhythmias

Supraventricular tachycardia

For patients with paroxysmal SVT (AVNRT, AVRT, AT) associated with syncope, catheter ablation is first-line therapy, if the patient is willing to undergo the procedure.[3] If the patient refuses, or catheter ablation is ineffective, medical therapy is warranted. The available classes of medication used for this purpose include AV nodal blocking agents (in the absence of preexcitation) or antiarrhythmic drugs. For atrial flutter, a decision regarding a rate control versus rhythm strategy is needed. For rate control, AV nodal blocking agents should be used. For a rhythm strategy, catheter ablation is preferred first-line therapy and antiarrhythmic drug therapy is an alternative. In patients with syncope and atrial fibrillation, the decision regarding catheter ablation, AV nodal blocking agents, or antiarrhythmic drug therapy should be individualized.[57,58]

Ventricular arrhythmias

For patients with syncope and polymorphic VT (torsades de pointe), treatment is immediate discontinuation of all QT interval prolonging drugs and correction of electrolyte abnormalities. The approach to a patient with syncope and ventricular arrhythmias is complex and highly depends on the underlying substrate. Options for treatment include catheter ablation, AV nodal blocking agents, or antiarrhythmic drug therapy.[4,21] In certain situations, patients who present with syncope should be considered for an implantable cardioverter defibrillator (ICD):

1. Syncope of undetermined origin with clinically relevant, hemodynamically significant sustained VT or ventricular fibrillation induced at EPS[59]
2. Unexplained syncope and nonischemic dilated cardiomyopathy with significant LV dysfunction[2,58,60]

3. Patients with hypertrophic cardiomyopathy with 1 or more recent episodes of syncope suspected to be arrhythmic in nature[61]
4. Patients with ARVC who present with syncope and documented sustained ventricular arrhythmias or of suspected arrhythmic cause[62–67]
5. ICD is recommended in patients with cardiac sarcoidosis presenting with syncope and documented spontaneous sustained ventricular arrhythmias. ICD is reasonable in patients with cardiac sarcoidosis and syncope suspected of arrhythmic cause, particularly if LV dysfunction is present or if there is a pacing indication.

The following indications for which ICD therapy may be reasonable or considered for patients with inherited primary arrhythmia syndromes[68]:

1. Brugada syndrome and either (1) spontaneous sustained VT with prior syncope or (2) spontaneous type 1 ECG pattern and syncope of suspected arrhythmic cause
2. Short-QT pattern and syncope of suspected arrhythmic cause
3. Long QT syndrome and suspected arrhythmic syncope who are on beta-blocker therapy or intolerant to beta-blocker therapy
4. CPVT and history of exercise or stress-induced syncope despite optimal medical therapy or left cervical sympathetic denervation
5. Early repolarization pattern and suspected arrhythmic syncope, or family history of early repolarization pattern with cardiac arrest.

REFERENCES

1. Shen W-K, Sheldon RS, Benditt DG, et al. 2017 ACC/AHA/HRS guideline for the evaluation and management of patients with syncope. J Am Coll Cardiol 2017;70(5).
2. Kusumoto FM, Schoenfeld MH, Barrett C, et al. 2018 ACC/AHA/HRS guideline on the evaluation and management of patients with bradycardia and cardiac conduction delay. Circulation 2018. [Epub ahead of print].
3. Page RL, Joglar JA, Caldwell MA, et al. 2015 ACC/AHA/HRS guideline for the management of adult patients with supraventricular tachycardia. Heart Rhythm 2016;13(4).
4. Al-Khatib SM, Stevenson WG, Ackerman MJ, et al. 2017 AHA/ACC/HRS guideline for management of patients with ventricular arrhythmias and the prevention of sudden cardiac death: a report of the American College of Cardiology/American Heart Association task force on clinical practice guidelines and the Heart Rhythm Society. J Am Coll Cardiol 2018;72(14):e91–220.
5. Alasti M, Machado C, Rangasamy K, et al. Pacemaker-mediated arrhythmias. J Arrhythmia 2018;34(5):485–92.
6. Sun BC, Emond JA, Camargo CA Jr. Characteristics and admission patterns of patients presenting with syncope to U.S. emergency departments, 1992-2000. Acad Emerg Med 2004;11:1029–34.
7. Birnbaum A, Esses D, Bijur P, et al. Failure to validate the San Francisco Syncope Rule in an independent emergency department population. Ann Emerg Med 2008;52:151–9.
8. Thiruganasambandamoorthy V, Stiell I, Wells G. Frequency and outcomes of syncope in the emergency department. Can J Emerg Med Care 2008;10:255–95.
9. McIntosh S, Da Costa D, Kenny RA. Outcome of an integrated approach to the investigation of dizziness, falls and syncope in elderly patients referred to a 'syncope' clinic. Age Ageing 1993;22:53–8.

10. Sud S, Klein GJ, Skanes AC, et al. Predicting the cause of syncope from clinical history in patients undergoing prolonged monitoring. Heart Rhythm 2009;6(2): 238–43.
11. Quinn J, Mcdermott D. Electrocardiogram findings in Emergency Department patients with syncope. Acad Emerg Med 2011;18(7):714–8.
12. Kapoor WN. Evaluation and outcome of patients with syncope. Medicine (Baltimore) 1990;69:160–75.
13. Krahn A, Subbiah R, Gula L, et al. Syncope: review of monitoring modalities. Curr Cardiol Rev 2008;4(1):41–8.
14. Dovgalyuk J, Holstege C, Mattu A, et al. The electrocardiogram in the patient with syncope. Am J Emerg Med 2007;25(6):688–701.
15. Marine JE. ECG Features that suggest a potentially life-threatening arrhythmia as the cause for syncope. J Electrocardiol 2013;46(6):561–8.
16. Quinn J, McDermott D, Stiell I, et al. Prospective validation of the San Francisco Syncope Rule to predict patients with serious outcomes. Ann Emerg Med 2006; 47:448–54.
17. Martin TP, Hanusa BH, Kapoor WN. Risk stratification of patients with syncope. Ann Emerg Med 1997;29:459–66.
18. Colivicchi F, Ammirati F, Melina D, et al. OESIL (Osservatorio Epidemiologico sulla Sincope nel Lazio) Study Investigators. Development and prospective validation of a risk stratification system for patients with syncope in the emergency department: the OESIL risk score. Eur Heart J 2003;24:811–9.
19. Del Rosso A, Ungar A, Maggi R, et al. Clinical predictors of cardiac syncope at initial evaluation in patients referred urgently to a general hospital: the EGSYS score. Heart 2008;94:1620–6.
20. Reed MJ, Newby DE, Coull AJ, et al. The ROSE (Risk stratification Of Syncope in the Emergency department) study. J Am Coll Cardiol 2010;55:713–21.
21. Brignole M, Moya A, De Lange F, et al. 2018 ESC guidelines for the diagnosis and management of syncope. Eur Heart J 2018;39(21):1883–948.
22. Costantino G, Casazza G, Reed M, et al. Syncope risk stratification tools vs clinical judgment: an individual patient data meta-analysis. Am J Med 2014;127. 1126.e13-25.
23. Sarasin FP, Junod AF, Carballo D, et al. Role of echocardiography in the evaluation of syncope: a prospective study. Heart 2002;88:363–7.
24. Recchia D, Barzilai B. Echocardiography in the evaluation of patients with syncope. J Gen Intern Med 1995;10:649–55.
25. Chiu DT, Shapiro NI, Sun BC, et al. Are echocardiography, telemetry, ambulatory electrocardiography monitoring, and cardiac enzymes in emergency department patients presenting with syncope useful tests? A preliminary investigation. J Emerg Med 2014;47:113–8.
26. Douglas PS, Garcia MJ, Haines DE, et al. ACCF/ASE/AHA/ASNC/HFSA/HRS/ SCAI/SCCM/SCCT/SCMR 2011 appropriate use criteria for echocardiography. A report of the American College of Cardiology Foundation Appropriate Use Criteria Task Force, American Society of Echocardiography, American Heart Association, American Society of Nuclear Cardiology, Heart Failure Society of America, Heart Rhythm Society, Society for Cardiovascular Angiography and Interventions, Society of Critical Care Medicine, Society of Cardiovascular Computed Tomography, and Society for Cardiovascular Magnetic Resonance. J Am Coll Cardiol 2011;57:1126–66.

27. Sparrow PJ, Merchant N, Provost YL, et al. CT and MR imaging findings in patients with acquired heart disease at risk for sudden cardiac death. Radiographics 2009;29:805–23.
28. Sparrow P, Merchant N, Provost Y, et al. Cardiac MRI and CT features of inheritable and congenital conditions associated with sudden cardiac death. Eur Radiol 2009;19:259–70.
29. Steckman DA, Schneider PM, Schuller JL, et al. Utility of cardiac magnetic resonance imaging to differentiate cardiac sarcoidosis from arrhythmogenic right ventricular cardiomyopathy. Am J Cardiol 2012;110:575–9.
30. Janardhanan R. Echocardiography in arrhythmogenic right ventricular dysplasia/cardiomyopathy: can the technology survive in the era of cardiac magnetic resonance imaging? Cardiol J 2015;22:355–6.
31. Woelfel AK, Simpson RJ Jr, Gettes LS, et al. Exercise-induced distal atrioventricular block. J Am Coll Cardiol 1983;2:578–81.
32. Linzer M, Yang EH, Estes NA 3rd, et al. Diagnosing syncope. Part 2: unexplained syncope. Clinical efficacy assessment project of the American College of Physicians. Ann Intern Med 1997;127:76–86.
33. Reiffel JA, Schwarzberg R, Murry M. Comparison of autotriggered memory loop recorders versus standard loop recorders versus 24-hour Holter monitors for arrhythmia detection. Am J Cardiol 2005;95:1055–9.
34. Bass EB, Curtiss EI, Arena VC, et al. The duration of Holter monitoring in patients with syncope. Is 24 hours enough? Arch Intern Med 1990;150:1073–8.
35. Sivakumaran S, Krahn AD, Klein GJ, et al. A prospective randomized comparison of loop recorders versus Holter monitors in patients with syncope or presyncope. Am J Med 2003;115:1–5.
36. Brown AP, Dawkins KD, Davies JG. Detection of arrhythmias: use of a patient-activated ambulatory electrocardiogram device with a solid-state memory loop. Br Heart J 1987;58:251–3.
37. Cumbee SR, Pryor RE, Linzer M. Cardiac loop ECG recording: a new noninvasive diagnostic test in recurrent syncope. South Med J 1990;83:39–43.
38. Locati ET, Moya A, Oliveira M, et al. External prolonged electrocardiogram monitoring in unexplained syncope and palpitations: results of the SYNARR-Flash study. Europace 2016;18:1265–72.
39. Schuchert A, Maas R, Kretzschmar C, et al. Diagnostic yield of external electrocardiographic loop recorders in patients with recurrent syncope and negative tilt table test. Pacing Clin Electrophysiol 2003;26:1837–40.
40. Barrett PM, Komatireddy R, Haaser S, et al. Comparison of 24-hour Holter monitoring with 14-day novel adhesive patch electrocardiographic monitoring. Am J Med 2014;127:95–7.
41. Turakhia MP, Hoang DD, Zimetbaum P, et al. Diagnostic utility of a novel leadless arrhythmia monitoring device. Am J Cardiol 2013;112:520–4.
42. Joshi AK, Kowey PR, Prystowsky EN, et al. First experience with a Mobile Cardiac Outpatient Telemetry (MCOT) system for the diagnosis and management of cardiac arrhythmia. Am J Cardiol 2005;95:878–81.
43. Rothman SA, Laughlin JC, Seltzer J, et al. The diagnosis of cardiac arrhythmias: a prospective multi-center randomized study comparing mobile cardiac outpatient telemetry versus standard loop event monitoring. J Cardiovasc Electrophysiol 2007;18:241–7.
44. Krahn AD, Klein GJ, Yee R, et al. Randomized assessment of syncope trial: conventional diagnostic testing versus a prolonged monitoring strategy. Circulation 2001;104:46–51.

45. Lombardi F, Calosso E, Mascioli G, et al. Utility of implantable loop recorder (Reveal Plus) in the diagnosis of unexplained syncope. Europace 2005;7:19–24.
46. Podoleanu C, DaCosta A, Defaye P, et al. FRESH investigators. Early use of an implantable loop recorder in syncope evaluation: a randomized study in the context of the French healthcare system (FRESH study). Arch Cardiovasc Dis 2014;107:546–52.
47. Sulke N, Sugihara C, Hong P, et al. The benefit of a remotely monitored implantable loop recorder as a first line investigation in unexplained syncope: the EaSyAS II trial. Europace 2016;18:912–8.
48. Linker NJ, Voulgaraki D, Garutti C, et al, PICTURE Study Investigators. Early versus delayed implantation of a loop recorder in patients with unexplained syncope–effects on care pathway and diagnostic yield. Int J Cardiol 2013;170: 146–51.
49. Edvardsson N, Frykman V, van Mechelen R, et al, PICTURE Study Investigators. Use of an implantable loop recorder to increase the diagnostic yield in unexplained syncope: results from the PICTURE registry. Europace 2011;13:262–9.
50. Gulamhusein S, Naccarelli GV, Ko PT, et al. Value and limitations of clinical electrophysiologic study in assessment of patients with unexplained syncope. Am J Med 1982;73:700–5.
51. Sagristà-Sauleda J, Romero-Ferrer B, Moya A, et al. Variations in diagnostic yield of head-up tilt test and electrophysiology in groups of patients with syncope of unknown origin. Eur Heart J 2001;22:857–65.
52. Gatzoulis KA, Karystinos G, Gialernios T, et al. Correlation of noninvasive electrocardiography with invasive electrophysiology in syncope of unknown origin: implications from a large syncope database. Ann Noninvasive Electrocardiol 2009;14:119–27.
53. Mehta D, Mori N, Goldbarg SH, et al. Primary prevention of sudden cardiac death in silent cardiac sarcoidosis: role of programmed ventricular stimulation. Circ Arrhythm Electrophysiol 2011;4:43–8.
54. Priori, et al. 2103 HRS/EHRA/APHRS Expert consensus statement of the diagnosis and management of patients with inherited primary arrhythmic syndromes.
55. Tracy CM, Epstein AE, Darbar D, et al. 2012 ACCF/AHA/HRS focused update of the 2008 guidelines for device-based therapy of cardiac rhythm abnormalities: a report of the American College of Cardiology Foundation/American Heart Association Task Force on Practice Guidelines and the Heart Rhythm Society. Circulation 2012;126:1784–800.
56. Epstein AE, DiMarco JP, Ellenbogen KA, et al. ACC/AHA/HRS 2008 guidelines for device-based therapy of cardiac rhythm abnormalities: a report of the American College of Cardiology/American Heart Association Task Force on practice guidelines (writing committee to revise the ACC/AHA/NASPE 2002 guideline update for implantation of cardiac pacemakers and antiarrhythmia devices). J Am Coll Cardiol 2008;51:e1–62.
57. January CT, Wann LS, Alpert JS, et al. 2014 AHA/ACC/HRS guideline for the management of patients with atrial fibrillation. J Am Coll Cardiol 2014;64(21).
58. Kirchhof P, Benussi S, Kotecha D, et al. 2016 ESC guidelines for the management of atrial fibrillation developed in collaboration with EACTS. Eur Heart J 2016; 37(38):2893–962.
59. Kusumoto FM, Calkins H, Boehmer J, et al. HRS/ACC/AHA expert consensus statement on the use of implantable cardioverter-defibrillator therapy in patients who are not included or not well represented in clinical trials. Circulation 2014; 130:94–125.

60. Zipes DP, Camm AJ, Borggrefe M, et al. ACC/AHA/ESC 2006 guidelines for management of patients with ventricular arrhythmias and the prevention of sudden cardiac death: a report of the American College of Cardiology/American Heart Association Task Force and the European Society of Cardiology Committee for practice guidelines (writing committee to develop guidelines for management of patients with ventricular arrhythmias and the prevention of sudden cardiac death). Circulation 2006;114:1088–132.
61. Gersh BJ, Maron BJ, Bonow RO, et al. 2011 ACCF/AHA guideline for the diagnosis and treatment of hypertrophic cardiomyopathy: a report of the American College of Cardiology Foundation/American Heart Association Task Force on Practice Guidelines. Developed in collaboration with the American Association for Thoracic Surgery, American Society of Echocardiography, American Society of Nuclear Cardiology, Heart Failure Society of America, Heart Rhythm Society, Society for Cardiovascular Angiography and Interventions, and Society of Thoracic Surgeons. Circulation 2011;124:e783–831.
62. Bhonsale A, James CA, Tichnell C, et al. Incidence and predictors of implantable cardioverter-defibrillator therapy in patients with arrhythmogenic right ventricular dysplasia/cardiomyopathy undergoing implantable cardioverter-defibrillator implantation for primary prevention. J Am Coll Cardiol 2011;58: 1485–96.
63. Bhonsale A, James CA, Tichnell C, et al. Risk stratification in arrhythmogenic right ventricular dysplasia/cardiomyopathy-associated desmosomal mutation carriers. Circ Arrhythm Electrophysiol 2013;6:569–78.
64. Corrado D, Leoni L, Link MS, et al. Implantable cardioverter-defibrillator therapy for prevention of sudden death in patients with arrhythmogenic right ventricular cardiomyopathy/dysplasia. Circulation 2003;108:3084–91.
65. Corrado D, Wichter T, Link MS, et al. Treatment of arrhythmogenic right ventricular cardiomyopathy/dysplasia: an international task force consensus statement. Circulation 2015;132:441–53.
66. Link MS, Laidlaw D, Polonsky B, et al. Ventricular arrhythmias in the North American multidisciplinary study of ARVC: predictors, characteristics, and treatment. J Am Coll Cardiol 2014;64:119–25.
67. Corrado D, Calkins H, Link MS, et al. Prophylactic implantable defibrillator in patients with arrhythmogenic right ventricular cardiomyopathy/dysplasia and no prior ventricular fibrillation or sustained ventricular tachycardia. Circulation 2010;122:1144–52.
68. Priori SG, Wilde AA, Horie M, et al. HRS/EHRA/APHRS expert consensus statement on the diagnosis and management of patients with inherited primary arrhythmia syndromes. J Arrhythmia 2014;30(1):1–28.

Inherited Cardiac Arrhythmias and Channelopathies

Jessica Kline, DO[a], Otto Costantini, MD[b],*

KEYWORDS

- Inherited cardiac arrhythmias • Channelopathies • Long QT syndrome
- Brugada syndrome • Short QT syndrome
- Catecholaminergic polymorphic ventricular tachycardia

KEY POINTS

- Inherited arrhythmias can cause sudden death in young and healthy individuals.
- A family history and an electrocardiogram are important clinical tools.
- With advances in genetic diagnostics, many diseases can be screened for.
- Several phenotypes have been linked to a specific genotype guiding pharmacologic management and device implantation.

INTRODUCTION

Sudden cardiac death (SCD) is responsible for approximately 300,000 deaths per year. A minority of these deaths occur in young healthy individuals. Over the last 3 decades, with advances in our understanding of genetic disease, we have begun to link clinical phenotypes to specific genotypes. Many of these unexplained sudden deaths occur owing to genetic mutations that affect the sodium (Na^+), potassium (K^+), and calcium (Ca^{2+}) channels responsible for ion transport across the myocardial cell membrane. If there is a loss or gain of function in one of these ion channels, the action potential is altered in ways that predispose the patient to life threatening arrhythmias. The disease that pioneered the era of genetic characterization of arrhythmic phenotypes is the long QT syndrome (LQTS) in the early to mid-1990s.[1] Since then several other high-profile disease phenotypes have been linked to specific genetic disorders of ion channels. Examples of such diseases include the short QT syndrome (SQTS), Brugada syndrome (BrS), and catecholaminergic polymorphic

Disclosure Statement: The authors have no financial relationships to disclose pertaining to the content of this article.
[a] Cardiovascular Disease, Summa Health System, 95 Arch Street, Suite 300, Akron, OH 44304, USA; [b] Cardiovascular Disease Fellowship, Summa Health Heart and Vascular Institute, Summa Health System, 95 Arch Street, Suite 350, Akron, OH 44304, USA
* Corresponding author.
E-mail address: costantinio@summahealth.org

ventricular tachycardia (VT). These inherited channelopathies affect approximately 1 in 3000 people, and may be responsible for a minority of deaths owing to sudden infant death syndrome (SIDS).

Many other diseases are being linked to specific genetic disorders. Examples are congenital heart block and inherited sinus node dysfunction. In addition, although beyond the scope of this article, many genes that predispose patients to familial cardiomyopathies also cause life-threatening arrhythmias, sometimes before the cardiomyopathy is manifest. The most common examples are hypertrophic cardiomyopathy and arrhythmogenic ventricular dysplasia.

Unfortunately, SCD or resuscitated cardiac arrest is often the initial symptom. However, a detailed look into the history of these patients reveals that many had prior symptoms or a family history of premature SCD that went unrecognized. It is imperative that the internist recognize a suspicious family history, obtain an electrocardiogram (ECG), and refer to a specialist when appropriate. These disease may lie dormant for years, but if recognized and diagnosed early they can be treated and patients and their families can be risk stratified.

LONG QT SYNDROME

LQTS is the most common of the inherited channelopathies and affects about 1 in 2000 people.[2,3] Arrhythmias occur owing to abnormal cardiac repolarization, which prolongs the QT corrected (QTc) interval and causes polymorphic VT (Torsades de Pointes), resulting in syncope or cardiac arrest. When first described, LQTS was characterized based on the mode of genetic transmission. The Romano-Ward syndrome was the most common, inherited in an autosomal dominant fashion. The Jervell and Lange-Nielsen syndrome, in contrast, was less common and inherited in an autosomal-recessive fashion. With the advent of genotyping, to date, 10 genes have been identified that correlate with 10 different syndromes.[2,4] LQTS genetic testing became commercially available in 2004 for LQT1, 2, 3, 5, and 6, with an approximately 75% yield when the patient has a clear clinical presentation.[1] Today genetic testing is available for all identified genes, with varying yields.

The specific genetic mutations encode ion channel subunits or proteins that regulate the ion channels affecting the different currents responsible for the action potential of myocardial cells primarily affecting repolarization and therefore prolonging the QT interval. The K^+ channel mutations result in a loss of function, which prolongs phase 3 of the action potential. The Na^+, Ca^{2+} channel mutation results in a gain of function, which causes persistent inward currents prolonging phases 0, 1, and 2 of the action potential. LQT1, LQT2, and LQT3 account for approximately 85% of cases.[4] The others have been rarely described in the literature. Each of the genotypes has a specific ECG pattern, clinical trigger, and response to therapy. Each of the genotypes is described in **Table 1**.

Clinical Presentation

LQTS is typically manifested in children or young adults, although it can occur from the first to the sixth decade of life.[5] It is recognized as a significant contributor to SIDS.[6] Patients can present with palpitation, near syncope, syncope, or cardiac arrest.

Unfortunately, patients are often misdiagnosed with vasovagal syncope owing to their young age.

The internist, as the physician who will first evaluate these patients, should recognize the difference between a benign presentation and a more malignant one. Because these syncopal or near syncopal episodes are a result brief runs of

Table 1
Genotypes of LQTS

Subtype	Gene	Chromosomal Locus	Ion Channel Affected	Mode of Transmission
LQT1	KCNQ1	11p 15.5	Decreased I_{Ks}	AD
LQT2	KCNH2	7q35-q36	Decreased I_{Kr}	AD5A
LQT3	SCN5A	3p21	Increased I_{Na}	AD
LQT4	ANK2	4q25-q27	Multiple	AD
LQT5	KCNE1	21q22.1-q22.2	Decreased I_{Ks}	AD
LQT6	KCNE2	21q22.1	Decreased I_{Kr}	AD
LQT7	KCNJ2	17q23.1-q24.2	Decreased I_{K1}	AD
LQT8	CACNA1C	12p13.3	Increased I_{Ca-L}	Sporadic
LQT9	CAV3	3p25	Increased I_{Na}	Sporadic
LQT10	SCN4B	11q23	Increased I_{Na}	—

Abbreviations: I_{Ca-L}, L-type Ca^{2+} current; I_{K1}, inward rectifier K^+ current; I_{Kr} rapid component of delayed rectifier K^+ current; I_{Ks}, slow component of delayed rectifier K^+ current; I_{Na}, Na^+ current.

polymorphic VT, they are brief, typically lasting seconds, and not associated with change in position. In fact they can often occur while sitting or driving. They are very different in nature from vagal, hypotensive events typically associated with an aura, a trigger, and often lasting several minutes to hours. Of course if they persist, they will degenerate into ventricular fibrillation (VF), causing SCD or a resuscitated cardiac arrest. An ECG is paramount in the diagnosis, although overlap of the QTc interval with normal subjects remains a clinical dilemma. The presence of a family history of unexplained SCD in a young, first-degree relative is also very important to ascertain. Patients have a 5% yearly risk of syncope or cardiac arrest. After the first episode of syncope, mortality increases to 20% in the first year and to more than 50% within 10 years if the LQTS continues to go unrecognized.[7] Advances in genetic testing have highlighted the fact that the ECG of asymptomatic, but genetically positive, patients can show normal QT intervals. This is due to the variable penetrance of many of the genes causing LQTS.[8]

Screening and Diagnosis

Approximately 50% of patients with LQTS will have a normal QTc interval, which underscores the role of genetic testing. It is recommended that LQTS be considered in any postpubertal female with QTc intervals of greater than 480 ms or any postpubertal male with a QTc of greater than 470 ms. Each QTc should be measured manually from either lead II or lead V_5 and calculated using Bazett's formula. A detailed clinical scoring system was developed by Moss and Schwartz to risk stratify patients (**Table 2**). It takes into account ECG parameters, clinical history, and family history. Any score of greater than 4 indicates a greater than 75% likelihood of a positive genetic testing result. That this scoring system is useful only for the index case and not for screening family members, who may have no clinical symptoms.[9] Other important ECG findings include T wave alternans, a sign of electrical instability, and notched T waves, which are a poor prognostic sign.

Risk Stratification

Key risk factors for a worse prognosis and a high risk of SCD include a QTc of greater than 500 ms, the presence of LQTS-related symptoms, LQT2 or LQT3 genotype, and

Table 2
Diagnostic criteria of LQTS

	Findings		Points
Electrocardiographic	Duration of QTc	>480 ms	3
		460–470 ms	2
		450 ms (in males)	1
	Torsades de Pointes		2
	T wave alternans		1
	Notched T wave in 3 leads		1
	Low heart rate for age		0.5
Clinical history	Syncope	With stress	2
		Without stress	1
	Congenital deafness		0.5
Family history	Family members with definite LQTS		1
	Unexplained SCD before the age of 30 y among immediate family members		0.5

Scoring: <1 point, low probability; 2–3 points, intermediate probability; >4 points, high probability.
Adapted from Schwartz PJ, Moss AJ, Vincent GM, et al. Diagnostic criteria for the long QT syndrome: An update. Circulation 1993;88(2):783; with permission.

female sex. The strongest of these predictors is the length of the QTc interval.[5] Patients who have had syncope before puberty or survive a cardiac arrest before age 7 have an overall worse prognosis.[10] If patients suffer from syncope or cardiac arrest in the first year of life and survive they are at a very high risk for recurrent events.[11] Beta-blockers (BBs) and implantable defibrillators can reduce overall risk to approximately 3% to 4% over 5 years. Asymptomatic but genetically positive patients have approximately a 10% risk between birth and 40 years of age of experiencing a life-threatening arrhythmia without therapy.[12] Male patients and those with LQT1 genotype are at a lower risk.

Management

There are no available placebo-controlled, randomized clinical trials regarding the management of LQTS. Management strategies have been primarily derived from large registries with data regarding BB and implantable cardioverter-defibrillator (ICD) therapy. ICD indications are detailed in **Box 1**. A single lead ICD is preferred especially given that these patients are young at implantation and are at high risk for lead complications over time. The subcutaneous ICD is a new exciting option that avoids many of the endovascular complications.

BB therapy is recommended for all patients less than 40 years of age who are symptomatic. The longer acting BB should be used to avoid fluctuations in blood levels, specifically nadolol and propranolol.[13] BB therapy should be continued after an ICD is implanted. In fact, owing to the adrenergic response after a delivered shock, a BB may avoid the risk of recurrent shocks. Patients should be counseled to avoid abrupt cessation of BBs, because this may precipitate events. BB therapy has proven beneficial in LQT1 and LQT2; however, data suggest it may be proarrhythmic in LQT3 where arrhythmias may be due to bradycardia. In LQT3, mexilitene may be useful because it inhibits the inward sodium current. Patients should be diligent to maintain adequate hydration and electrolyte replacement, particularly in the setting of vomiting, diarrhea, or excessive sweating. They should also avoid all medications that can cause QT prolonging or any medication that can deplete potassium or magnesium.

> **Box 1**
> **Indications for ICD in LQTS**
>
> - Aborted cardiac arrest as secondary prevention
> - Recurrent cardiac arrest despite optimal medical therapy
> - Intolerance to primary pharmacotherapy (BB)
> - Symptomatic patients with QTc of 500 ms or greater, especially women with LQT2
> - LQT3 genotype

Advanced therapy using left cardiac sympathetic denervation is reserved for patients with high-risk features and in whom an ICD is contraindicated or refused or in patients in whom BB therapy is ineffective, not tolerated, or contraindicated.

Indications for Genetic Testing

Asymptomatic patients with unequivocal or unexplained QT prolongation should be considered for genetic testing. Patients with suspected LQTS on the basis of symptoms should also be tested, regardless of the baseline QTc interval. All first-degree relatives of a genotype-positive index case should be tested. If any of these relatives test positive, their first-degree relatives should be tested in a concentric pattern. Any patient who has had drug-induced Torsades de Pointes should be evaluated regardless of the baseline resting QTc interval. Although controversial, most cases with SIDS should undergo postmortem genetic testing.

Long QT Syndrome 1

LQT1 is the most common genotype accounting for 30% to 35% of all LQTS cases. It is caused by a loss of function mutation in the KCNQ1 gene, which encodes the slowly activating delayed rectifier K^+ current. This mutation causes slowing of repolarization, prolongation of phase 3 of the action potential and, as a result, prolongation of the QT interval. It typically manifests around 5 to 15 years of age and is triggered by physical or emotional stressors, such as swimming or diving. With exercise stress testing and increased heart rate, the QTc interval fails to shorten and often prolongs further. Thus, polymorphic VT is a tachy-mediated phenomenon. The ECG shows broad-based T waves. Approximately 37% of patients with LQT1 will have normal resting QTc intervals.[12] Beta-blockade is extremely effective and patients do not commonly need an ICD.

Long QT Syndrome 2

LQT2 accounts for approximately 25% to 30% of LQTS patients and occurs owing to a mutation in the KCNH2 gene that encodes the rapidly activating component of the K^+ current.[14] Onset is typically at puberty and symptoms are often triggered by loud auditory stimuli. Polymorphic VT typically occurs as a result of a pause, thus the short–long–short phenomenon. The ECG demonstrates low amplitude or notched T waves, which are associated with a higher risk for arrhythmic events.[15] With this genotype, women in the first 6 months postpartum are at higher risk for SCD events.[16] Beta-blockade is only moderately effective in this genotype, and an ICD is used more commonly.

Long QT Syndrome 3

LQT3 only accounts for about 5% to 10% of cases. It is caused by a mutation in the SCN5A gene that causes prolonged activation of the Na^+ channel, thus prolonging repolarization. It occurs at puberty or later and usually at rest or during sleep, making it particularly lethal. It has a worse prognosis than LQT1 or LQT2. The ECG demonstrates a long ST isoelectric segment with normal T wave morphology. Approximately 10% of patients have a normal QT interval.[12] Sodium channel blockers such as mexilitene may be beneficial, but caution is recommended because this agent could exacerbate BrS[17] because this mutation can also cause the BrS.[18] BB therapy has no beneficial effect.

Rare Forms of Long QT Syndrome

Several other rare genetic abnormalities have been identified that are linked to phenotypic syndromes associated with specific clinical and ECG features. Anderson–Tawil syndrome, Timothy's syndrome, and the Jervell and Lange Nielsen syndrome are 3 examples. They are often associated with extracardiac manifestations, underscoring the fact that genes that encode the ion channel proteins also encode proteins outside of the cardiac system. These syndromes are rare, they remain poorly understood, and a detailed discussion is beyond the scope of this article.

SHORT QT SYNDROME

The SQTS was first described clinically in 2000. Since then, 3 subtypes have been discovered that are inherited in an autosomal-dominant fashion. They are the result of a gain-of-function mutation in the K^+ channels genes, which results in shortened phase 3 repolarization.[19] Mutations in the same genes that result in a loss of function prolong repolarization and are responsible for LQTS variants. Unlike LQTS, this is an extremely rare disorder with very high mortality. Patients suffer from both atrial and ventricular arrhythmias.[20–22] It is diagnosed by recognition of a QTc 330 ms or less.

Clinical Presentation

Patients present with a mean age of 30 years, but SCD death is described between the ages of 3 months and 77 years of age. Symptoms include palpitations, syncope, or cardiac arrest. Patients also often present with paroxysmal atrial fibrillation.

Screening and Diagnosis

The diagnosis of SQTS criteria has been a matter of debate. Gollob and colleagues[23] have attempted to set forth a scoring scheme similar to LQTS but it has not been widely accepted. Agreed upon criteria for diagnosis include a QTc of 330 ms of less (or a QTc of ≥360 ms with a known pathogenic mutation), a family history of SQTS, a family history of SCD at 40 years old or younger, or survival of a cardiac arrest with a structurally normal heart. The ECG demonstrates tall symmetric peaked T waves and often a type 1 BrS pattern.[24,25]

Management and Prognosis

The number of reported cases is small and therefore the treatment and management is poorly defined. It is recommended that every patient with SQTS receive an ICD, especially those who have survived cardiac arrest or have had a prior syncopal episode. Quinidine has shown promise in treatment by prolonging the QTc interval and decreasing the amplitude of the T wave.[26]

CATECHOLAMINERGIC POLYMORPHIC VENTRICULAR TACHYCARDIA

Catecholaminergic polymorphic VT is an autosomal-dominant genetic mutation that causes exercise or stress-induced syncope or SCD in the setting of a structurally normal heart. The hallmark of this disease is the bidirectional VT also seen with digitalis toxicity.[27,28] The genetic abnormality is a mutation of the cardiac ryanodine receptor (RYR2), which controls the Ca^{2+} release in the sarcoplasmic reticulum. The mutation causes cellular calcium overload and triggers delayed after depolarizations that cause VT. It accounts for 10% to 15% of SIDS and is present in 35% of autopsy-negative SCD.

Clinical Presentation

Patients present in the first or second decades of life and episodes of palpitation, near syncope, or syncope are initiated by physical or emotional stress. A positive family history of exercise induced syncope, seizures, or SCD is present in 30% of cases. Patients will commonly present with bidirectional VT.

Screening and Diagnosis

The ECG is unremarkable. Exercise stress testing is crucial in the diagnosis and prognosis. As patients exercise and the heart rate exceeds 110 to 130 bpm, premature ventricular contractions start to occur. With continued exercise they will develop bigeminy, polymorphic, or bidirectional VT, and occasionally VF. Supraventricular tachycardias may occur. Loop recorders or Holter monitoring can be helpful. Electrophysiology studies are not useful because the ventricular arrhythmias are not inducible. The administration of isoproterenol or epinephrine may be useful in those who cannot exercise, including very young patients and postarrest patients.

Management and Prognosis

Nadolol and other long-acting BB have been effective in preventing VT and should be titrated to the highest tolerated dose. Despite BB use, 30% of patients will still have VT.[29] Therefore, any patient who survives a cardiac arrest should have an ICD placed. Patients with an ICD need to continue on BB therapy to avoid VT storm after an ICD shock. If a shock occurs, amiodarone, lidocaine, and magnesium have all been proven effective acutely to decrease further shocks. A small study showed that flecainide in addition to BB may be helpful in reducing ventricular arrhythmia burden.[30] Catheter ablation of bidirectional VT has shown promise but experience is limited.[31] A poor prognosis is typical in patients diagnosed in childhood, those not treated with BB therapy, and persistence of complex ectopy with exercise testing despite treatment. A thorough clinical history and genetic testing are indicated in first-degree relatives. Genetically positive family members should undergo exercise stress testing and should initiate BB therapy even if stress testing is negative.

BRUGADA SYNDROME

The BrS is another inherited channelopathy that predisposes patients to the risk of arrhythmic SCD. It is characterized by spontaneous or drug-induced ST elevation in the right precordial leads (V1–V3) associated with ventricular conduction delay. Three electrocardiographic types have been delineated.[32,33] The syndrome has a higher prevalence in Southeast Asian countries and descendants of those countries. It is unclear why an Asian prevalence exists, but some investigators suspect it is related to an Asian-specific sequence in the promoter region of SCN5A. A total of 12 genes have been reported to be pathologic. They cause either a decrease in inward Na^+ or

Ca^{2+} currents or an increase in the outward K^+ current. Genotypes that affect the Na^+ channel account for approximately 33% of patients. The mean age at presentation is 40 years old, but the syndrome has been described in patients between the ages of 2 months and 77 years.

Clinical Presentation

Patients present with VF or aborted SCD, syncope, nocturnal agonal respirations, palpitations, and chest discomfort that occurs at rest or during sleep. They can also occur during a febrile state or with vagotonic conditions, but only rarely during exercise. It is not uncommon that SCD is the initial presentation. Family history of SCD may be present, but does not predict the risk of arrhythmic events.

Screening and Diagnosis

The ECG of the type I syndrome demonstrates ST segment elevation with a typical coved pattern in V1 to V3 and a descending ST segment. Often there is evidence of diffuse conduction delay with prolonged PR and QRS intervals. ST elevation occurs spontaneously or after a drug challenge with procainamide, ajmaline, or flecainide. The sensitivity of the drug challenge is unknown, but is estimated to be approximately 77%.[33] An electrophysiological study usually demonstrates evidence of conduction disease and inducible ventricular arrhythmias. BrS occurs in patients without structural heart disease. However, postmortem studies and endomyocardial biopsies have shown evidence of fibrosis and fatty infiltration.[34,35] **Box 2**, derived from the Heart Rhythm Society/European Heart Rhythm Association/Asia-Pacific Heart Rhythm Society Expert Consensus Statement on the Diagnosis and Management of Inherited Primary Arrhythmias,[36] describes the criteria for diagnosis of BrS.

Risk Stratification

Any patient that survived a VF arrest or with syncope and an ECG consistent with spontaneous type I pattern should undergo permanent cardiac defibrillator

---

Box 2
Criteria for diagnosis of Brugada syndrome

Symptomatic patients
- Type I ST segment elevation via drug challenge or spontaneously in at least 1 right precordial lead (V_1 or V_2).

In asymptomatic patients
- Attenuation of the ST segment in peak exercise followed by coved ST segment elevations at rest.
- Atrial fibrillation.
- Absence of structural heart disease.
- ST-T alternans, spontaneous left bundle branch block, or premature ventricular contractions during prolonged ECG monitoring.
- Presence of first-degree atrioventricular block and left axis deviation.
- Ventricular Effective Refractory Period (ERP) of less than 200 ms during an electrophysiology study.
- Signal averaged ECG with late potentials.
- Fragmented QRS.

Data from Priori SG, Wilde AA, Horie M, et al. HRS/EHRA/APHRS expert consensus statement on the diagnosis and management of patients with inherited primary arrhythmia syndromes. Heart Rhythm 2013;10:1932–1963.

placement.[37] Other high-risk factors include male gender, atrial fibrillation, or a fragmented QRS. There is no consensus on the use of electrophysiologic study to risk stratify patients. Importantly, the PRogrammed ELectrical stimUlation preDictive valuE (PRELUDE) registry showed that the inability to induce arrhythmias does not correlate with a negative predictive value.[38] A family history of SCD and the presence of an SCN5A mutation have proven to be high risk predictors as well.[39–41]

Management and Prognosis

The ICD is the only proven effective therapeutic strategy for the prevention of SCD in BrS. If patients are asymptomatic they should not have an ICD placed on the basis of family history of SCD alone. Pharmacotherapy has been directed toward the outward potassium channels or inward sodium and calcium channels. Isoproteronol increases L-type calcium channel function and has been useful to treat VT storm. Quinidine blocks the outward K^+ channel and inward sodium channels and has been shown to prevent induction of VF and suppress spontaneous ventricular arrhythmias. Catheter ablation may be useful in high-risk patients with an ICD and recurrent appropriate ICD shocks. Genetic testing should be done in all first-degree relatives if the index case has an abnormal genotype. Genetic testing should not be used if patients do not have ECG findings.

CONGENITAL HEART BLOCK

There are 2 types of third-degree atrioventricular (AV) block, acquired and congenital. Congenital heart block occurs in 2 forms. In the first form, it is often diagnosed in utero owing to fetal bradycardia. This is due to an embryologic disorder and abnormal formation of the AV node or His-Purkinje system. In the other form, the conduction system forms normally, but it is attacked by the mother's anti-Rho antibodies, which pass through the placenta. Mortality is approximately 50% in a fetus and 5% to 15% in newborns.

Screening and Diagnosis

Typically congenital heart block is found during prenatal testing. A complete biophysical profile should be completed to avoid a rushed delivery as a result of bradycardia. Newborns should be monitored for heart failure as a result of AV block. Third-degree AV block is occasionally found in older asymptomatic children with a structurally normal heart.

Management and Prognosis

Indications for pacing include pauses of more than 3 seconds, heart failure, junctional instability or wide QRS escape rhythms, declining exercise performance, QT prolongation, and complex ventricular ectopy. Newborns require an epicardial pacing system.

INHERITED SINUS NODE DYSFUNCTION

The sinus node plays a critical role in the generation of the electrical impulse. Its function and unique action potential is due to specific ion channels. Impairment of the sinus node is typically acquired, but in some cases a genetic cause is responsible. The implicated genes include the NA, the pacemaker (HCN), and Ca channels. Defects in regulatory proteins and calcium-handling proteins are also involved.[42]

Screening and Diagnosis

Diagnosis depends on noninvasive testing. Bradycardias are typically out of proportion for age. Sinus pauses of more than 3 seconds are common. Patients should have an ECG and at least 24 hours of ambulatory monitoring. Exercise stress testing shows evidence of chronotropic incompetence. Symptomatic patients should be treated with a permanent pacemaker.

REFERENCES

1. Keating M, Atkinson D, Dunn C, et al. Linkage of a cardiac arrhythmia, the long QT syndrome, and the Harvey ras-1 gene. Science 1991;252:704–6.
2. Roden DM. Clinical practice. Long-QT syndrome. N Engl J Med 2008;358: 169–76.
3. Schwartz PJ, Stramba-Badiadle M, Crotti L, et al. Prevalence of the congenital Long QT Syndrome. Circulation 2009;120:1761–7.
4. Wilde AA, Tan HL. Inherited arrhythmia syndromes. Circ J 2007;71:A12–9.
5. Zipes DP, Camm AJ, Borggrefe M, et al. ACC/AHA/ESC 2006 guidelines for management of patients with ventricular arrhythmias and the prevention of sudden cardiac death: a report of the American College of Cardiology/American Heart Association Task Force and the European Society of Cardiology Committee for Practice Guidelines (Writing Committee to develop guidelines for management of patients with ventricular arrhythmias and the prevention of sudden cardiac death). J Am Coll Cardiol 2006;48:e247–346.
6. Schwartz PJ, Stramba-Badiale M, Segantini A, et al. Prolongation of the QT interval and the sudden infant death syndrome. N Engl J Med 1998;338:1709–14.
7. Roden DM, Lazzara R, Rosen M, et al. Multiple mechanisms in the long-QT syndrome. Current knowledge, gaps, and future directions. The SADS Foundation task force on LQTS. Circulation 1996;94:1996–2012.
8. Priori SG, Napolitano C, Schwartz PJ. Low penetrance in the long-QT syndrome: clinical impact. Circulation 1999;99:529–33.
9. Schwartz PJ, Moss AJ, Vincent GM, et al. Diagnostic criteria for the long QT syndrome. An update. Circulation 1993;88:782–4.
10. Priori SG, Napolitano C, Schwartz PJ, et al. Association of long QT syndrome loci and cardiac events among patients treated with beta-blockers. JAMA 2004;292: 1341–4.
11. Spazzolini C, Mullally J, Moss AJ, et al. Clinical implications for patients with long QT syndrome who experience a cardiac event during infancy. J Am Coll Cardiol 2009;54:832–7.
12. Priori SG, Schwartz PJ, Napolitano C, et al. Risk stratification in the long QT syndrome. N Engl J Med 2003;348:1866–74.
13. Chockalingam P, Crotti L, Girardengo G, et al. Not all beta-blockers are equal in the management of long QT syndrome types 1 and 2: higher recurrence of events under metoprolol. J Am Coll Cardiol 2012;60:2092–9.
14. Curran ME, Splawski I, Timothy KW, et al. A molecular basis for cardiac arrhythmia: HERG mutations cause long QT syndrome. Cell 1995;80:795–803.
15. Malfatto G, Beria G, Sala S, et al. Quantitative analysis of T wave abnormalities and their prognostic implications in the idiopathic long QT syndrome. J Am Coll Cardiol 1994;23:296–301.
16. Seth R, Moss AJ, McNitt S, et al. Long QT syndrome and pregnancy. J Am Coll Cardiol 2007;49(10):1092.

17. Schwartz PJ, Priori SG, Locati EH, et al. Long QT syndrome patients with mutations of the SCN5A and HERG genes have differential responses to Na. Circulation 1995;92:3381–6.
18. Tan HL. Sodium channel variants in heart disease: expanding horizons. J Cardiovasc Electrophysiol 2006;17:S151–7.
19. Gaita F, Giustetto C, Bianchi F, et al. Short QT syndrome: a familial cause of sudden death. Circulation 2003;108:965–70.
20. Antzelevitch C, Francis J. Congenital short QT syndrome. Indian Pacing Electrophysiol J 2004;4:46–9.
21. Giustetto C, Di Monte F, Wolpert C, et al. Short QT syndrome: clinical findings and diagnostic-therapeutic implications. Eur Heart J 2006;27:2440–7.
22. Viswanathan MN, Page RL. Short QT: when does it matter? Circulation 2007;116: 686–8.
23. Gollob MH, Redpath CJ, Roberts JD. The short QT syndrome: proposed diagnostic criteria. J Am Coll Cardiol 2011;57:802–12.
24. Antzelevitch C, Pollevick GD, Cordeiro JM, et al. Loss of function mutations in the cardiac calcium channel underlying a new clinical entity characterized by St segment elevation, short QT intervals and sudden cardiac death. Circulation 2007;115:442–9.
25. Priori SG, Cerrone M. Genetic arrhythmias. Ital Heart J 2005;6:241–8.
26. Gaita F, Giustetto C, Bianchi F, et al. Short QT syndrome: pharmacological treatment. J Am Coll Cardiol 2004;43:1494–9.
27. Leenhardt A, Lucet V, Denjoy I, et al. Catecholaminergic polymorphic ventricular tachycardia in children. A 7–year follow-up of 21 patients. Circulation 1995;91: 1512–9.
28. Mohamed U, Napolitano C, Priori SG. Molecular and electrophysiological bases of catecholaminergic polymorphic ventricular tachycardia. J Cardiovasc Electrophysiol 2007;18:791–7.
29. Hayashi M, Denjoy I, Extramiana F, et al. Incidence and risk factors for arrhythmic events in catecholaminergic polymorphic ventricular tachycardia. Circulation 2009;119:2426–34.
30. Van der Werf C, Kannankeril PJ, Sacher F, et al. Flecainide therapy reduces exercise-induced ventricular arrhythmias in patients with catecholaminergic polymorphic ventricular tachycardia. J Am Coll Cardiol 2011;57:2244–54.
31. Kaneshiro T, Naruse Y, Nogami A, et al. Successful catheter ablation of bidirectional ventricular premature contractions triggering ventricular fibrillation in catecholaminergic polymorphic ventricular tachycardia with RyR2 mutation. Circ Arrhythm Electrophysiol 2012;5:e14–7.
32. Mizusawa Y, Wilde AA. Brugada syndrome. Circ Arrhythm Electrophysiol 2012;5: 606–16.
33. Rossenbacker T, Priori SG. The Brugada syndrome. Curr Opin Cardiol 2007;22: 163–70.
34. Coronel R, Casini S, Koopmann TT, et al. Right ventricular fibrosis and conduction delay in a patient with clinical signs of Brugada syndrome: a combined electrophysiological, genetic, histopathologic, and computational study. Circulation 2005;112:2769–77.
35. Frustaci A, Priori SG, Pieroni M, et al. Cardiac histological substrate in patients with clinical phenotype of Brugada syndrome. Circulation 2005;112:3680–7.
36. Priori SG, Wilde AA, Minoru H, et al. HRS/EHRA/APHRS expert consensus statement on the diagnosis and management of patients with inherited primary arrhythmia syndromes. Heart Rhythm 2013;10:1932–63.

37. Antzelevitch C, Brugada P, Borggrefe M, et al. Brugada syndrome: report of the second consensus conference. Heart Rhythm 2005;2:429–40.
38. Priori SG, Gasparini M, Napolitano C, et al. Risk stratification in Brugada syndrome: results of the PRELUDE (PRogrammed ELectrical stimUlation preDictive valuE) registry. J Am Coll Cardiol 2012;59:37–45.
39. Priori SG, Napolitano C, Gasparini M, et al. Natural history of Brugada syndrome: insights for risk stratification and management. Circulation 2002;105:1342–7.
40. Eckardt L, Probst V, Smits JP, et al. Long-term prognosis of individuals with right precordial ST-segment-elevation Brugada syndrome. Circulation 2005;111: 257–63.
41. Gehi AK, Duong TD, Metz LD, et al. Risk stratification of individuals with the Brugada electrocardiogram: a meta-analysis. J Cardiovasc Electrophysiol 2006;17: 577–83.
42. Milanesi R, Bucchi A, Baruscotti M. The genetic basis for inherited forms of sinoatrial dysfunction and atrioventricular node dysfunction. J Interv Card Electrophysiol 2015;43:121–34.

Antiarrhythmic Drugs
Risks and Benefits

Pranav Mankad, MD[a], Gautham Kalahasty, MD[b],*

KEYWORDS

- Antiarrhythmic therapy • Cardiac action potential • Mechanisms of arrhythmia
- Practical approach to antiarrhythmics

KEY POINTS

- Antiarrhythmic drugs continue to have an important role in the management of atrial and ventricular arrhythmias.
- Most antiarrhythmic drugs have no proven mortality benefit when administered on a chronic basis, requiring a careful risk/benefit analysis.
- The side effects and proarrhythmic effects of antiarrhythmic drugs are distinct concepts and are critical to the risk/benefit analysis.
- Antiarrhythmic drugs can be safely used for symptomatic relief and prophylaxis of most cardiac arrhythmias.

INTRODUCTION

The narrow therapeutic window of antiarrhythmic drugs (AADs) and their potential for lethal proarrhythmia pose a unique clinical challenge without parallel in medical practice.[1] The therapeutic window of some of these medications overlaps significantly with their proarrhythmic effect. It is for this reason that the concept of *proarrhythmia* should be distinguished from that of a *side effect*. Side effects of AADs can be cardiac or extracardiac, but are due to mechanisms unrelated to their targeted ion channel. An example of a cardiac side effect of an AAD is the negative inotropic effect of disopyramide (Norpace), potentially exacerbating heart failure. Disopyramide also has extracardiac side effects resulting in constipation, dry mouth, and urinary retention because of its anticholinergic properties. However, it is its proarrhythmic effect of potentially causing torsades de pointes (TdP) that should be respected the most because such proarrhythmia can cause sudden cardiac arrest. Proarrhythmias occur primarily

---

Disclosure Statement: None.
a Department of Cardiology, Virginia Commonwealth University Health System, PO Box 980053, Richmond, VA 23235, USA; b Department of Electrophysiology, Virginia Commonwealth University Health System, PO Box 980053, Richmond, VA 23235, USA
* Corresponding author.
E-mail address: gautham.kalahasty@vcuhealth.org

Med Clin N Am 103 (2019) 821–834
https://doi.org/10.1016/j.mcna.2019.05.004
0025-7125/19/© 2019 Elsevier Inc. All rights reserved.

because of the effects on ion channels, not only at toxic levels but also at therapeutic levels. Drug-drug interactions can also alter the metabolism of an AAD or potentiate its effect, such that a previously therapeutic dose may become toxic. Because of their proarrhythmic effects, some AADs need to be started on an inpatient basis. For example, dofetilide can only be initiated on an inpatient basis (manufacturer recommendation and standard practice) with continuous telemetry monitoring and serial electrocardiograms to monitor the QT interval. Some cardiologists will initiate sotalol on an outpatient basis with close follow-up. With current ablation techniques, most atrial and ventricular arrhythmias can be potentially treated (cured or palliated) without the need for antiarrhythmic medications. However, atrial fibrillation and ventricular tachycardia (VT) in a structurally abnormal heart remain difficult to cure. In addition, not all patients are candidates for ablation. It is therefore often critical to weigh the risks and benefits of antiarrhythmic medications in such cases. Although primary care physicians will often defer to cardiologists or electrophysiologists for the management of AADs, it is nevertheless important for all clinicians to have a basic understanding of these powerful drugs. This understanding starts with cellular electrophysiology.

CARDIAC ACTION POTENTIAL

Fig. 1 demonstrates the action potential (AP) of a ventricular myocardial cell. There are some differences in AP phases and their slopes in other cardiac cells. However, ventricular myocardial cells are used as standard models because they contain all phases of an AP and are illustrative of the main concepts. The following is a simplified explanation of an AP.

Depolarization

*From the resting membrane potential, any ion shift that makes the membrane more positive will result in depolarization: Phase 0 in **Fig. 1**. (ECG correlate: QRS interval)*

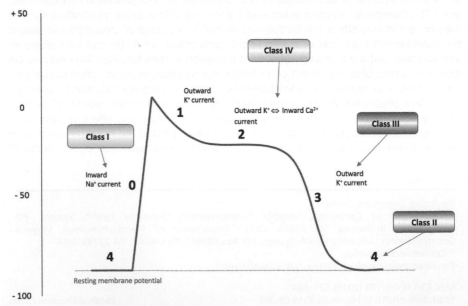

Fig. 1. Action potential in ventricular myocyte.

The cardiac myocyte in an equilibrium state is normally polarized between −80 and −95 mV.[2] While in phase 4, if the resting membrane potential is brought to threshold, a rapid influx of Na^+ ions flow into the cell via voltage-gated sodium-ion channels, generating phase 0 of the AP as demonstrated in **Fig. 1**.

Repolarization

After depolarization, any ion shifts that make the membrane more negative will result in repolarization. This includes phases 1, 2, and 3 (see **Fig. 1**). (ECG correlate: QT interval)

During phase 1 there is transient outward potassium current via I_{To} channels, which begins the repolarization process. The density of I_{To} channels is different between endocardium/epicardium and different chambers of the heart.

Phase 2 is characterized by a plateau (see **Fig. 1**). During this phase there is balance between outward current caused by late-activating calcium channels (L-type Ca channels) and inward potassium current, which results transiently in a net neutral membrane potential.

Phase 3 (see **Fig. 1**) is characterized by rapid repolarization caused by inward potassium currents (I_{Kr}, I_{Ks}). Toward the end of phase 3 there is activation of inward rectifying potassium current (I_{K1}), which brings the membrane potential close to the resting membrane potential.

Electrical Diastole

Phase 4 or resting membrane potential is maintained by I_{K1}. In the pacemaker cells (ie, the sinus node) there is spontaneous depolarization toward membrane threshold, resulting in AP generation. β-Blockers can reduce the slope of this phase.

ARRHYTHMIA MECHANISMS

There are 3 mechanisms for cardiac arrhythmias: Re-entry, abnormal automaticity, and triggered activity.

1. Re-entry is the by far most common mechanism of arrhythmia and does not require abnormal cellular electrophysiology. For re-entry to occur a propagating impulse needs to encounter an area of resistance—anatomic (due to scar) or functional (due to heterogeneity in electrophysiologic properties of the myocardium). In addition, there needs to be unidirectional block in one limb of the circuit (due to refractoriness) and propagation of the impulse along another limb (**Fig. 2**A). If the initially refractory limb of the circuit has recovered, the impulse can travel retrogradely along that limb. This circuit can perpetuate when the impulse returns to the original bifurcation point and finds the anterograde limb excitable again. This can result in circus movement tachycardia (re-entry) (**Fig. 2**B).
   - The spatial excitable gap is the amount of tissue that is available to be depolarized in a re-entry circuit.[3]
   - AADs that work by increasing refractoriness (class III) shorten the excitable gap and therefore increase the likelihood that a propagating impulse would find the tissue refractory and, therefore, unable to sustain a re-entrant tachyarrhythmia (**Fig. 2**C).[4,5]
   - Some AADs slow the conduction velocity by decreasing the slope of phase 0 of AP (class I, and especially class IC drugs), creating areas of slow conduction in the presence of an anatomic (scar) or a functional conduction barrier. This can also occur in healthy tissue, resulting in proarrhythmia with a mechanism of re-entry (**Fig. 2**D).[1]

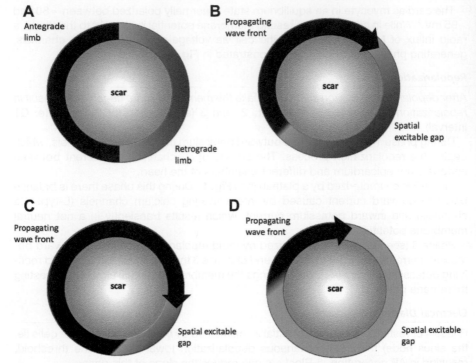

Fig. 2. Mechanism of action of antiarrhythmic drug in re-entry. (*A*) Re-entry substrate. (*B*) Schematic of re-entry mechanism. (*C*) Class III agents increase refractoriness and decrease excitable gap. (*D*) Class IC agents decrease conduction velocity and increase excitable gap.

2. Abnormal automaticity occurs when a group of cells gain the ability to spontaneously depolarize during electrical diastole (phase 4 of AP) and reach membrane threshold, resulting in an AP. Pacemaker cells of the heart (SA node, AV node, Purkinje cells) demonstrate this phenomenon inherently.[3] Pathologic examples of arrhythmias resulting from this mechanism include multifocal atrial tachycardia and some idiopathic VTs.

3. Triggered activity is due to afterdepolarizations, abnormal depolarizations that occur during the repolarization phase. If a cardiac cell reaches membrane threshold again, an extrasystole occurs. A tachyarrhythmia results when these extrasystoles perpetuate. There are 2 types of afterdepolarizations.
   - Early afterdepolarization, which occurs during phase 2 or 3 of AP. This mechanism is responsible for long QT-related arrhythmias such as polymorphic VT or TdP.
   - Late afterdepolarization occurs once the myocyte has been repolarized but before another AP would normally occur (early phase 4). This occurs because of intracellular calcium overload, resulting in ventricular premature beats that in turn can serve to trigger VT or ventricular fibrillation. This mechanism is involved in tachyarrhythmias seen during digoxin toxicity, catecholaminergic polymorphic ventricular tachycardia (CPVT), and ischemia-induced ventricular arrhythmias.[3]

CLASSIFICATION AND CLINICAL PEARLS

The modified Vaughan-Williams classification system of antiarrhythmic drugs is based on their primary effect on phases of AP and remains the most practical approach to understand their clinical use. However, many of these drugs can affect more than one type of ion channel, both at therapeutic doses and especially at toxic doses. This classification system does not include adenosine or digoxin despite their widespread use in the management of arrhythmias. Only the most commonly used AADs are discussed herein and only some clinical pearls are emphasized. The reader is referred to a more comprehensive discussion of these drugs. Although not part of the Vaughan-Williams classification, adenosine and digoxin have important roles in the treatment of arrhythmias and are also discussed below.

Class I: Sodium-Channel Blockers

These drugs affect phase 0 of AP, which results in prolongation of depolarization (widening of the QRS complex) and slowing of conduction. There are three subgroups according to their different pharmacokinetic properties.

IA: quinidine, procainamide, and disopyramide

Along with sodium-channel blocking properties, these drugs also have moderate potassium-channel blocking activity, which results in prolonged repolarization and long QTc ("The Sicilian Gambit"). Because of its I_{To} blocking properties, quinidine has a niche role in suppressing ventricular arrhythmias in Brugada syndrome.[6] These medications suppress myocardial contractility and therefore can result in exacerbation of congestive heart failure. Procainamide can be used in atrial fibrillation with rapid ventricular response in the setting of Wolf-Parkinson-White (WPW) syndrome. Its effects include termination of atrial fibrillation and slowing of conduction through the accessory pathway. N-Acetylprocainamide (NAPA; a metabolite of procainamide) can cause prolonged QT and TdP.[5] There are no large-scale outcome trials for these agents, and their effect on mortality is neutral at best. Their use is becoming very uncommon, as is their availability.

IB: lidocaine and mexiletine

These drugs have higher affinity for inactivated sodium channels (depolarized state) and are therefore more effective with tachyarrhythmias (use-dependent pharmacokinetics). Lidocaine is more effective at ischemic sites and is therefore useful in treating ventricular arrhythmias associated with acute myocardial infarction. It is not used for prophylaxis of ventricular arrhythmias and has no role in the treatment of supraventricular tachycardia (SVT). Lidocaine levels are monitored closely because of its narrow therapeutic window. Extracardiac side effects include severe central nervous system toxicity including tonic-clonic seizures and altered mental status. Mexiletine is an oral medication that is structurally related to lidocaine and is used for prophylaxis of ventricular arrhythmias. It is used as an adjunct to class III antiarrhythmics (such as amiodarone) for treatment of refractory VT. It is rarely used as monotherapy and is associated with gastrointestinal and central nervous system side effects.[2]

IC: flecainide and propafenone

These drugs are powerful inhibitors of fast sodium channels, resulting in decreased slope of phase 0 of the AP. However, they can also inhibit the rapid repolarization current I_{Kr}, resulting in QRS widening and slowing of conduction through the His-Purkinje system. Propafenone also has some β-blocker effects. Seven percent of white patients have a genetic absence of a hepatic cytochrome enzyme (P-450 2D6) resulting in slow metabolism of propafenone and, therefore, an increase of its β-blocker effect. Class IC antiarrhythmics show use-dependent pharmacokinetics. At faster heart rates there are more sodium channels in open or inactivated state, and these AADs have higher affinity for sodium channels in this state. As a result, monomorphic VT can occur at faster heart rates. It is prudent to conduct a stress test on patients started on these drugs to rule out this important proarrhythmic effect. This is also the mechanism by which atrial fibrillation can organize into a relatively slow atrial flutter (1C Flutter). Rapid conduction of the atrial flutter through the AV node in 1:1 fashion results in very fast ventricular activation with unusual intraventricular aberration (wide QRS complex), owing to propafenone's use-dependent kinetics and its effect on I_{Kr} channels. Therefore, these drugs should always be used in conjunction with AV nodal blockers to slow AV nodal conduction.[7] The CAST (Cardiac Arrhythmia Suppression Trial—flecainide) and CASH (Cardiac Arrest Study Hamburg—ropafenone) studies profoundly influenced the use of AADs by demonstrating increased mortality from these drugs owing to the proarrhythmic risk in patients with structural heart disease.[1,8] The proarrhythmia is due to their heterogenic electrical effects on healthy myocytes versus areas of scar or surrounding slow conduction, potentially setting up the substrate for ventricular re-entry (see **Fig. 2**C).[4] As a result of these studies, they are absolutely contraindicated in patients with coronary disease and a low left ventricular ejection fraction.

Class II

β-Blockers
The antiarrhythmic effect of β-blockers is more complicated than just their antiadrenergic effects. In acute myocardial infarction, the antiadrenergic effects result in decreased levels of cyclic AMP, reducing the risk of ventricular fibrillation. Catecholamines can potentiate arrhythmias via any of the 3 mechanisms described earlier in this article. β-blockers are generally effective in any tachyarrhythmia (SVT or VT) associated with increased sympathetic β-adrenergic tone. In patients with VT storm, that is, refractory to antiarrhythmics and ablation, sympathetic denervation to the heart via stellate ganglion blockade or bilateral cardiac sympathetic denervation via surgical approach can be effective and further provides evidence for the role of the sympathetic nervous system as a trigger for tachyarrhythmias.[9] β-Blockers depress activity of the SA node, AV node, and ectopic foci. They also increase AV node effective refractory period and can thus affect both anterograde and retrograde AV nodal conduction.

Class III

Potassium-channel blockers: amiodarone, dronedarone, sotalol, ibutilide, dofetilide
This class of medications blocks potassium channels and lengthens AP duration and effective refractory periods. The prolongation of the AP duration manifests on the surface ECG as a prolonged QT interval.

Amiodarone and sotalol are "mixed" class III agents because of their additional effects beyond potassium-channel blockade. Amiodarone has class I effects by inhibiting inactive sodium channels at high heart rates. It also noncompetitively binds at β-adrenergic receptors and even has some mild class IV effects. As remarkable as amiodarone is with its myriad of electrophysiologic effects, it is also remarkable for its many side effects and toxicities. The extracardiac side-effect profile is much higher than its risk of serious proarrhythmia. As a result, although the most effective antiarrhythmic available, amiodarone should be used with caution, especially in a young population. A meta-analysis of amiodarone trials established amiodarone as neutral with respect to mortality and as low risk in regard to proarrhythmia, supporting its use in patients with congestive heart failure and cardiomyopathies.[10] Initiation of low-dose amiodarone in an outpatient setting for atrial arrhythmias is common. However, some experts recommend inpatient monitoring for initiation with large loading doses. Amiodarone is among the most widely prescribed AADs for both atrial and ventricular arrhythmias. As such, close monitoring for side effects is mandatory. Most side effects are related to the cumulative dose and can sometimes be reversible when the drug is discontinued. A complete discussion of the side effects of amiodarone is beyond the scope of this article. Amiodarone is capable of affecting virtually every organ system including the lungs (pulmonary fibrosis, acute respiratory distress syndrome), the thyroid gland (hypo- and hyperthyroidism), the gastrointestinal tract (liver, gastrointestinal distress), the eyes (corneal microdeposits, optic neuritis, photosensitivity), the skin (bluish discoloration), and the neurologic system (tremors). Although thyroid toxicity is more common, pulmonary toxicity is among the most feared complications of amiodarone therapy because it is often nonreversible and potentially fatal. Acute lung injury/acute respiratory distress syndrome and diffuse alveolar hemorrhage is rare but is associated with up to a 50% mortality rate. Risk factors for this include recent cardiothoracic surgery, high Fio_2 (fraction of inspired oxygen), and pulmonary angiography. The occurrence of severe, irreversible interstitial pulmonary fibrosis may be as high as 1.2%. It is related to the cumulative dose administered and the dose intensity. The overall mortality of interstitial pulmonary fibrosis is 9%. Milder forms of lung toxicity have been reported in the range of 4.2% to 17% of patients. For example, lipoid pneumonia, which is sometimes referred to as the "amiodarone effect," is mostly asymptomatic and recognized only by mild declines in lung diffusion capacity. This occurs as a result of the lipophilic moiety of amiodarone causing it to concentrate in organs with high lipid content (liver and lung).[11] Most of these conditions are reversible, and symptoms improve with drug withdrawal.

Dronedarone is a noniodinated congener of amiodarone used to maintain sinus rhythm in patients with atrial fibrillation. Because of the lack of iodine molecules, dronedarone has less pulmonary and thyroid toxicity. Like amiodarone, it primarily has class III effects but also has class II and IV effects. It is contraindicated in symptomatic heart failure or in permanent atrial fibrillation and should not be used as an agent for rate control.[12,13] It is not approved for the treatment of ventricular tachyarrhythmias. On the other hand, amiodarone is approved by the Food and Drug Administration for the treatment of life-threatening ventricular arrhythmias, but not for atrial tachyarrhythmias. Compared with other antiarrhythmic drugs, polymorphic VT (TdP) is less common with amiodarone and dronedarone, likely because of their homogeneous effect on all myocardial cells and channels.[4]

Sotalol (Betapace) has important class II effects in addition to its class III effects. At doses less than 160 mg/d, its class III effects are not evident. Ibutilide (an intravenous drug), dofetilide (Tikosyn), and sotalol demonstrate reverse-use dependence; their effect is more pronounced at lower heart rates, resulting in increased risk of TdP with sinus bradycardia. This is especially concerning in patients receiving sotalol because of its additional β-blocker effects. Because of the high risk of TdP from QT prolongation, dofetilide and sotalol should be initiated with in-hospital electrocardiographic QTc monitoring.[14] The proarrhythmic risk of dofetilide and sotalol increases with concomitant QT-prolonging medications or with renal dysfunction. Both drugs are renally excreted and can lead to fatal proarrhythmias if their use is continued in patients with acute renal failure. Dose-adjusted use in mild to moderate renal dysfunction is possible if creatinine is stable.

Class IV

The calcium-channel blockers verapamil and diltiazem are nondihydropyridine calcium-channel blockers. Their antiarrhythmic properties are achieved primarily through increasing the refractory period of the AV node, and are mainly used to control the ventricular rate during atrial fibrillation and for termination and prevention of SVTs dependent on the AV node. Calcium-channel blockers are contraindicated in heart failure with reduced ejection fraction. Verapamil is the drug of choice for idiopathic VT, Belhassen type.[15]

Digoxin

Digoxin blocks sodium-potassium ATPase, ultimately leading to increased intracellular calcium, which results in increased inotropy. It enhances vagal tone and results in inhibition of SA node and AV node. It has a narrow therapeutic window and can precipitate toxicity in the setting of renal dysfunction. The common manifestations of an increased level are nausea, vomiting, diarrhea, and changes in color vision. At toxic levels digoxin can cause paroxysmal atrial tachycardia with AV block, bidirectional VT, or high-degree AV block. Digoxin is considered safe in pregnancy and is widely used in pediatric patients with tachyarrhythmias.[16] The clinical uses of digoxin for the treatment of arrhythmias in adults has largely been supplanted by the use of β-blockers and calcium-channel blockers.

Adenosine

Adenosine opens adenosine-sensitive inward rectifier potassium channels, resulting in inhibition of the sinus and AV node. Adenosine also shortens the atrial refractory period heterogeneously across atrial myocardium and therefore can trigger atrial fibrillation in as many as 10% of patients who receive it.[17] Because it has a mild effect on ventricular myocardium, ventricular ectopy can also be seen immediately following administration. Patients with active bronchospasm may experience severe and persistent bronchoconstriction. Adenosine should not be given to patients with reactive airway disease. Patients who have undergone autologous heart transplantation have a hypersensitivity to adenosine and should not receive adenosine in doses in excess of 3 mg or even at all. Its transient effect on the AV node makes it an ideal choice for treatment of SVT, including SVT associated with WPW syndrome. However, it is absolutely contraindicated in patients with WPW and atrial fibrillation (pre-excited atrial fibrillation) because it can potentially lead to more rapid conduction of atrial fibrillation to the ventricles via the accessory pathway by selectively inhibiting the AV node, resulting in ventricular fibrillation. Adenosine can be safely given to pregnant patients.

ANTIARRHYTHMICS IN CLINICAL PRACTICE

With the advancement of ablation therapy, the need for AADs has certainly waned. For most SVTs, atrial flutter, and idiopathic VT in structurally normal hearts, ablation is often offered as first-line therapy because the cure rates are extremely high. For atrial fibrillation or VT in ischemic or nonischemic cardiomyopathies, ablation is usually offered as second-line therapy after failure of at least one AAD. AADs still have an important role in the management of acute arrhythmias when a patient is not a candidate for ablation, when ablation is not successful, or when the patient prefers a more conservative approach. Based on the preceding discussion, the decision to initiate an AAD requires careful consideration of the risks and benefits. In some cases, the desire to treat an arrhythmia is based on symptom relief rather than expected mortality benefit. With the exception of β-blockers none of the antiarrhythmic medications can claim a mortality benefit. For example, in patients with minimally symptomatic atrial fibrillation and adequate rate control, the chronic use of amiodarone may not be justified. If an AAD is to be prescribed chronically, a complete discussion highlighting toxicities and proarrhythmic risks should be carried out with the patient. The approach to the use of AADs in atrial fibrillation is now discussed in more depth.

The most important factors to consider in choosing an AAD are as follows.

Arrhythmia Origin and Mechanism

The origin and mechanism of the arrhythmia being treated is important in selecting an AAD. If the arrhythmia is supraventricular in origin such as SVT, SVT associated with WPW syndrome, atrial fibrillation, atrial flutter, or atrial tachycardia, the choice of AAD (depending on acuity of arrhythmia, presence or absence of structural heart disease, and patient comorbidities) include a wide range of options (**Table 1**). If the arrhythmia is ventricular in origin such as monomorphic VT, polymorphic VT, ventricular fibrillation, or frequent PVCs, the choice of AADs might include procainamide, quinidine, lidocaine, mexiletine, sotalol, and amiodarone. (see **Table 1**).[18] In some cases the origin of the arrhythmia may be known but not the mechanism (re-entry versus triggered versus enhanced automaticity). Specific AADs may be the drug of choice for specific arrhythmias with known mechanisms. Flecainide has a niche role in CPVT in combination with β-blockers. CPVT is an inherited disorder that results in mutations affecting proteins that regulate intracellular calcium levels in cardiac muscle cells, resulting in calcium overload and ventricular arrhythmias in a structurally normal heart that lead to sudden cardiac death. Ibutilide is the drug of choice in atrial fibrillation with WPW syndrome (pre-excited atrial fibrillation). Adenosine, β-blockers and calcium-channel blockers have a role in treatment of some idiopathic VTs (VT in a structurally normal heart): adenosine in outflow tract VT, β-blockers in outflow tract VT and CPVT, and verapamil in fascicular VT.[19]

Arrhythmia Acuity and Chronicity

The pattern of occurrence, acuity, and chronicity of the arrhythmia also play a role in AAD selection. Electrical cardioversion is the treatment of choice for symptomatic,

Table 1 Medications by arrhythmia type		
	Atrial Arrhythmias	Ventricular Arrhythmias
Adenosine	Yes	Idiopathic VT
Digoxin	Yes	No
β-Blocker (II)	Yes	Idiopathic VT
Calcium-channel blockers (IV)	Yes	Idiopathic VT
Procainamide, quinidine (IA)	Yes	Yes
Disopyramide (IA)	Yes	No
Lidocaine, mexiletine (IB)	No	Yes
Flecainide (IC)	Yes	Flecainide in CPVT
Propafenone (IC)	Yes	No
Dofetilide, ibutilide (III)	Yes	No
Sotalol, amiodarone (III)	Yes	Yes

Abbreviation: CPVT, catecholaminergic polymorphic ventricular tachycardia.

unstable patients with VT or SVT. **Table 2** describes the AADs that can be used in intravenous and oral forms.

- Re-entry SVTs can occur in an episodic pattern ranging from rare events to weekly or even daily episodes. For rare episodes, β-blockers or calcium-channel blockers can be prescribed as needed for acute termination as an outpatient. Along with adenosine, they can also be given on an intravenous basis for acute termination in an inpatient or emergency room setting. They can also be taken on a daily basis for prophylaxis against frequent episodes. Clinical judgment and a discussion with the patient are needed to decide when to initiate daily therapy, mostly dependent on the patient's quality of life.
- Intravenous β-blockers and intravenous calcium-channel blockers are often used for rate control in the setting of atrial tachyarrhythmias such as atrial fibrillation and atrial tachycardia. β-Blockers also blunt sympathetic response and can decrease the slope of phase 4 of the AP, which decreases automaticity and can potentially facilitate termination of atrial tachycardia and atrial fibrillation.
- Adenosine has a very short half-life (<10 s) as it is rapidly absorbed by red blood cells and vascular endothelium and metabolized very quickly. As a result, adenosine is only used acutely in the setting of narrow complex regular tachycardia. It can be both diagnostic and therapeutic. There are also rare adenosine-sensitive, idiopathic VTs. The effect of adenosine can be potentiated by pretreatment with β-blockers or calcium-channel blockers.
- Ibutilide is only available in intravenous formulation and is used to chemically cardiovert atrial fibrillation or flutter. However, it requires close telemetry monitoring for 4 hours immediately following administration given the risk of QT prolongation and TdP.[14] Pretreatment with ibutilide can facilitate electrical cardioversion.
- Intravenous amiodarone, procainamide, and lidocaine can be used for treatment of VT. Intravenous amiodarone and procainamide can also be used in the acute management of atrial fibrillation.
- Oral digoxin is used less commonly because of its limited efficacy and the availability of better alternatives. However, it can be modestly effective in the setting of atrial fibrillation with rapid ventricular rate in hospitalized patients with severe cardiomyopathy, hypotension, and normal renal function. Chronic outpatient administration of digoxin for rate control of atrial fibrillation is only modestly effective for patients in a resting state.

Table 2 Medications by acuity	
Acute Use (Intravenous)	**Chronic Use (Oral)**
Adenosine	
Digoxin	Digoxin
β-Blockers	β-Blockers
CCBs	CCBs
Procainamide (IA)	Quinidine (IA), disopyramide (IA)
Lidocaine (IB)	Mexiletine (IB) Flecainide (IC), propafenone (IC)
Ibutilide (III), amiodarone (III)	Sotalol (III), dofetilide (III), amiodarone (III)

Abbreviation: CCBs, calcium-channel blockers.

Structural Heart Disease

Structural heart disease is one of the most important determinants for AAD selection. For the purposes of AAD selection, structural heart disease is defined as the presence of coronary artery disease, significant cardiomyopathy, or any condition that causes myocardial fibrosis and scar (eg, sarcoid, hypertrophic cardiomyopathy, arrhythmogenic right ventricular dysplasia). The proarrhythmic potential of AADs is greater in patients with structural heart disease. Class IC AADs in particular are contraindicated in the presence of structural heart disease, especially coronary artery disease.[1] An ischemic workup is advisable before starting a class IC AAD in patients with multiple risk factors for coronary disease and in whom occult ischemia could be present.

Clinical Factors and Drug Monitoring

Comorbidities, concurrent medication use, and age also have an important impact on selection of AADs. The most critical comorbid conditions to be considered are chronic or acute kidney disease, liver function abnormalities, and chronic lung conditions. These conditions increase the risk of proarrhythmia and side effects.

- *Renal failure*. Digoxin, dofetilide, ibutilide, sotalol, and procainamide are renally cleared from the body and therefore cannot be used in patients with renal failure. In the presence of mild to moderate but stable renal dysfunction, dofetilide and sotalol may be given with dose adjustments. However, these patients often develop electrolyte abnormalities, which can potentiate the proarrhythmic risk of AADs. Close and frequent monitoring is required.
- *Hepatic dysfunction*. AADs that cannot be used in liver failure are amiodarone, procainamide, lidocaine, propafenone, flecainide, and disopyramide.
- *Heart failure* with reduced ejection fraction is an important comorbidity to consider when choosing an AAD. Patients with heart failure frequently experience both atrial and ventricular arrhythmias.
  - Class IA AADs (procainamide, quinidine, and disopyramide) suppress myocardial contractility and are contraindicated in heart failure.
  - Dronedarone is contraindicated in patients with New York Heart Association functional class II or, worse, congestive heart failure.
  - Calcium-channel blockers such as diltiazem and verapamil are also contraindicated in heart failure with reduced ejection fraction.
- Because many AADs are either metabolized by or inhibit cytochrome P450 enzymes in the liver, it is important to review a patient's medications and the interaction with AADs. For example, amiodarone interaction with warfarin results in increased serum concentration of warfarin and requires warfarin dose reduction to achieve the desired therapeutic level.

ATRIAL FIBRILLATION

Atrial fibrillation is one of the most commonly encountered arrhythmias. Its varied presentations and associated comorbidities make it an ideal arrhythmia on which to apply the concepts presented in this article. Virtually all of the antiarrhythmic medications discussed in this article (except lidocaine, mexiletine, and adenosine) have been used in some capacity or another for the management of atrial fibrillation. The pattern of atrial fibrillation occurrence, the severity of symptoms, the associated comorbidities, and the presence or absence of structural heart disease are all factors to be taken into account when selecting an AAD. **Fig. 3** presents an algorithm for drug selection based on these factors. If there is no structural heart disease, first-line

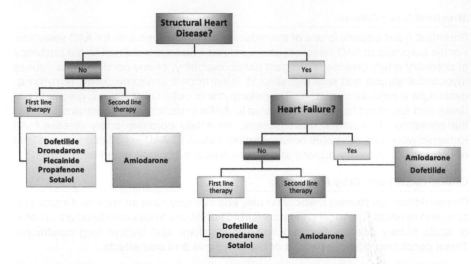

Fig. 3. Approach to selection of antiarrhythmic therapy in atrial fibrillation. (*Modified from* January CT, Wann LS, Alpert JS, et al. 2014 AHA/ACC/HRS guideline for the management of patients with atrial fibrillation: a report of the American College of Cardiology/American Heart Association Task Force on Practice Guidelines and the Heart Rhythm Society. J Am Coll Cardiol 2014;64:e1–76.)

antiarrhythmic therapy includes class III antiarrhythmics (except amiodarone) and class IC antiarrhythmics. Amiodarone is considered a second-line agent because of its side-effect profile. However, if the patient has other comorbidities such as renal failure, amiodarone may be the only appropriate choice. Chronic administration of any of these medications assumes a significant atrial fibrillation burden with symptoms. Nonpharmacologic therapies should also be considered. Propafenone and flecainide can be used as a "pill-in-the-pocket" approach. When the patient experiences a persistent episode of atrial fibrillation, they can be used for the acute cardioversion to sinus rhythm in the outpatient setting. If a patient has structural heart disease, the class IC antiarrhythmics are contraindicated.[20] In patients with rare (once a year) episodes and concurrent structural heart disease with congestive heart disease, periodic electrical cardioversion may be preferable to antiarrhythmic drugs. Finally, if the frequency of atrial fibrillation increases, dofetilide and amiodarone are the only suitable pharmacologic options because sotalol and dronedarone have been shown to increase mortality in patients with heart failure.[13,21]

SUMMARY

Despite the widespread availability and effectiveness of radiofrequency ablation, antiarrhythmic medications will continue to have an important role in the treatment of atrial and ventricular arrhythmias. Understanding arrhythmia mechanisms and the mechanism of action of antiarrhythmic drugs is the first step in being able to appropriately select an AAD. The Vaughan-Williams classification remains the most clinically practical method to classify antiarrhythmic medications. Recognizing the proarrhythmic potential and side-effect profile of each of the AADs is critical for their safe use. Shared decision-making practices and close clinical monitoring of patients is required. Because both atrial and ventricular arrhythmias have similar mechanisms, multiple AADs can be used for both. Individualized therapy based on the acuity of arrhythmia, the presence of underlying structural heart disease, the patient's comorbidities, and side-effect profile of the AAD dictate the choice. It is apparent from this discussion that the principle of "do no harm" is the overarching theme when using AADs. There are no data to confer a mortality benefit with the chronic use of AADs (except β-blockers). Their use can only be justified if they provide symptomatic relief without adverse effects.

REFERENCES

1. Echt DS, Liebson PR, Mitchell LB, et al. Mortality and morbidity in patients receiving encainide, flecainide, or placebo. N Engl J Med 1991;324(12):781–8.
2. Arnsdorf MF. The cellular basis of cardiac arrhythmias. A matrical perspective. Ann N Y Acad Sci 1990;601:263–80.
3. Antzelevitch C, Burashnikov A. Overview of basic mechanisms of cardiac arrhythmia. Card Electrophysiol Clin 2011;3(1):23–45.
4. Kowey PR, Marinchak RA, Rials SJ, et al. Pharmacologic and pharmacokinetic profile of class III antiarrhythmic drugs. Am J Cardiol 1997;80(8A):16G–23G.
5. The Sicilian gambit. A new approach to the classification of antiarrhythmic drugs based on their actions on arrhythmogenic mechanisms. Task Force of the Working Group on Arrhythmias of the European Society of Cardiology. Circulation 1991;84(4):1831–51.
6. Belhassen B, Glick A, Viskin S. Efficacy of quinidine in high-risk patients with brugada syndrome. Circulation 2004;110(13):1731–7.
7. Khan IA. Oral loading single dose flecainide for pharmacological cardioversion of recent-onset atrial fibrillation. Int J Cardiol 2003;87(2–3):121–8.
8. Kuck KH, Cappato R, Siebels J, et al. Randomized comparison of antiarrhythmic drug therapy with implantable defibrillators in patients resuscitated from cardiac arrest: the Cardiac Arrest Study Hamburg (CASH). Circulation 2000;102(7):748–54.
9. Podrid PJ, Fuchs T, Candinas R. Role of the sympathetic nervous system in the genesis of ventricular arrhythmia. Circulation 1990;82(2 Suppl):I103–13.
10. Vassallo P, Trohman RG. Prescribing amiodarone. JAMA 2007;298(11):1312.
11. Papiris SA, Triantafillidou C, Kolilekas L, et al. Amiodarone. Drug Saf 2010;33(7):539–58.
12. Connolly SJ, Camm AJ, Halperin JL, et al. Dronedarone in high-risk permanent atrial fibrillation. N Engl J Med 2011;365(24):2268–76.
13. Køber L, Torp-Pedersen C, McMurray JJV, et al. Increased mortality after dronedarone therapy for severe heart failure. N Engl J Med 2008;358(25):2678–87.
14. Stambler BS, Wood MA, Ellenbogen KA, et al. Efficacy and safety of repeated intravenous doses of ibutilide for rapid conversion of atrial flutter or fibrillation. Ibutilide Repeat Dose Study Investigators. Circulation 1996;94(7):1613–21.
15. Belhassen B, Rotmensch HH, Laniado S. Response of recurrent sustained ventricular tachycardia to verapamil. Br Heart J 1981;46(6):679–82.
16. Chow T, Galvin J, McGovern B. Antiarrhythmic drug therapy in pregnancy and lactation. Am J Cardiol 1998;82(4A):58I–62I.
17. Tokuda M, Matsuo S, Isogai R, et al. Adenosine testing during cryoballoon ablation and radiofrequency ablation of atrial fibrillation: a propensity score-matched analysis. Heart Rhythm 2016;13(11):2128–34.
18. Santangeli P, Rame JE, Birati EY, et al. Management of ventricular arrhythmias in patients with advanced heart failure. J Am Coll Cardiol 2017;69(14):1842–60.

19. Prystowsky EN, Padanilam BJ, Joshi S, et al. Ventricular arrhythmias in the absence of structural heart disease. J Am Coll Cardiol 2012;59(20):1733–44.

20. January CT, Wann LS, Alpert JS, et al. 2014 AHA/ACC/HRS guideline for the management of patients with atrial fibrillation: executive summary. Circulation 2014; 130(23):2071–104.

21. Waldo AL, Camm AJ, deRuyter H, et al. Effect of d-sotalol on mortality in patients with left ventricular dysfunction after recent and remote myocardial infarction. The SWORD Investigators. Survival With Oral d-Sotalol. Lancet 1996;348(9019):7–12.

Pharmacologic and Nonpharmacologic Management of Atrial Fibrillation

Vishal Dahya, MD[a], Tyler L. Taigen, MD[b],*

KEYWORDS

- Atrial fibrillation • Pharmacologic management • Catheter ablation
- Antiarrhythmic drugs

KEY POINTS

- Atrial fibrillation (AF) is the most commonly encountered arrhythmia, affecting approximately 3 million US patients.
- AF is defined by disorganized, rapid electric signaling and activation of the atria with associated irregular ventricular heart rates.
- Fundamentally, management of atrial fibrillation may be organized into risk stratification and/or treatment of heart failure, stroke prevention, and symptom control.

Atrial fibrillation (AF) is the most commonly encountered arrhythmia, affecting approximately 3 million US patients.[1] AF is characterized by disorganized, rapid electrical activity in the atria with associated irregular ventricular heart rates. AF may lead to rapid ventricular conduction, often associated with hemodynamic instability. In addition, as the atria fibrillate, blood pooling increases the risk of thromboembolic events and stroke.[1,2] AF is further defined by the cause of the arrhythmia. Valvular AF occurs in the setting of a mechanical heart valve, rheumatic mitral stenosis, or mitral valve repair. Nonvalvular AF includes all other causes. Numerous clinical risk factors and disease states predispose patients to AF. These include age, hypertension, thyroid disease, lung disease, sleep apnea, serious illness or infection, structural heart disease, and heart failure. In addition, the duration of AF classifies patients into important clinical subtypes as defined in **Table 1**.[1–3]

Disclosure Statement: The authors have no financial relationships to disclose pertaining to the content of this article.

[a] Cardiovascular Disease, Summa Health System, NEOMED University, Akron City Hospital, 95 Arch Street, Suite 300, Akron, OH 44304, USA; [b] Section of Pacing and Electrophysiology, Department of Cardiovascular Medicine, Heart and Vascular Institute, Cleveland Clinic Foundation, 9500 Euclid Avenue/J2, Cleveland, OH 44195, USA

* Corresponding author.

E-mail address: taigent@ccf.org

Table 1
Classifications of atrial fibrillation

Type of AF	Definition
Valvular AF	AF occurring in the setting of a mechanical or bioprosthetic aortic valve, rheumatic mitral stenosis, or mitral valve repair
Paroxysmal AF	AF that terminates spontaneously within 7 d of onset
Persistent AF	AF that is continuous and sustains >7 d
Long-standing persistent AF	AF that is continuous and >12 mo in duration
Permanent AF	Chronic AF, in which patient and clinician have decided that restoration of sinus rhythm is no longer an option

Fundamentally, management of AF can be divided into 2 main issues:

1. Risk stratification and anticoagulation for stroke prevention
2. Symptom control.

Stroke prevention and anticoagulation are beyond the scope of this article. (See Drs Viwe Mtwesi and Guy Amit's article, "Stroke Prevention in Atrial Fibrillation: The Role of Oral Anticoagulation," in this issue.) At the core of symptom control, treatment is tailored to either allow AF to continue with controlled heart rates, so-called rate control, versus restoring and maintaining sinus rhythm or rhythm control. Rate control strategies use atrioventricular (AV) nodal blockers to slow the ventricular rates and in turn diminish symptoms. On the other hand, rhythm control therapies aim to restore sinus rhythm acutely with pharmacologic or direct current (DC) cardioversion, and long-term with antiarrhythmic medications, or with endovascular catheter or surgical ablation therapies.[2,3]

RATE VERSUS RHYTHM CONTROL

A rate control strategy is most appropriate for asymptomatic patients with structurally and functionally normal hearts. In such patients, clinical trials have demonstrated that adequate rate control results in fewer hospitalization and improved hemodynamics and diastolic filling. Rate versus rhythm control strategies have been extensively evaluated in several randomized trials. The largest and most influential were the Atrial Fibrillation Follow-Up Investigation of Rhythm Management (AFFIRM)[4] and the Rate Control versus Electrical Cardioversion for Persistent Atrial Fibrillation (RACE).[5]

The AFFIRM trial was the first trial to directly compare rate control versus rhythm control. The trial enrolled more than 4000 subjects with nonvalvular AF and randomized them to a rate control or a rhythm control arm. The rate control group included therapeutic targets for heart rate and used AV nodal blockers, such as beta blockers, calcium channel blockers (CCBs), and digoxin. The rhythm control group used antiarrhythmic agents (class 1A, 1C, and III) in conjunction with cardioversion, as needed, to restore and maintain sinus rhythm. Anticoagulation therapy with warfarin was used in both groups. However, in the rhythm control group, warfarin could be stopped at the physician's discretion if sinus rhythm was maintained for at least 3 months. Subjects were followed for nearly 5 years. The trial found no statistically significant difference in the primary endpoint of overall mortality. Importantly, there were trends suggesting increased mortality (24% vs 21%) and ischemic stroke (7.1% vs 5.5%) in the rhythm control arm. The higher stroke risk in the rhythm control arm was attributed to interrupted anticoagulation therapy in subjects with presumed maintenance of sinus rhythm.[4] Moreover, subsequent studies have concluded that the trend toward increased mortality in the rhythm control group was likely secondary to the proarrhythmic effects associated with antiarrhythmic drugs (AADs). Although the study design has been criticized for selection bias, specifically because subjects with more prominent symptoms were often not enrolled to avoid randomization to rate control, it remains a landmark clinical trial. Decades after publication, results and interpretation of the AFFIRM trial continue to inform the understanding of the importance of stroke prevention and the difficulties associated with the use of antiarrhythmic medications.

The RACE study randomized subjects with persistent recurrent AF after cardioversion to rate control or rhythm control groups. More than 500 subjects were randomized and anticoagulated with warfarin with an international normalized ratio goal of 2 to 3. Rate control was achieved with AV nodal blockers such as beta blockers, digoxin, or calcium channel blocker. Rhythm control was achieved with electrical cardioversion, as needed, and long-term antiarrhythmic therapy with sotalol. As in the AFFIRM trial, results suggested that rate control was noninferior to rhythm control for the prevention of cardiovascular morbidity and mortality, and, therefore, may be appropriate for patients with recurrent arrhythmias following electrical cardioversion. Moreover, rates of thromboembolic events were higher in the rhythm control arm, primarily as a result of subtherapeutic anticoagulation.[5] A main concern limiting the clinical usefulness of the results observed in the RACE study was that the mean age of subjects was 68 years and, therefore, the applicability of rate control in younger patients remained unclear. Finally, contemporary interpretation of the AFFIRM and RACE trials must take into account that these studies were conducted before the widespread use of catheter-based ablation for rhythm control. Technologic advancement and improved safety and efficacy outcomes have positively affected patients treated with rhythm control using this procedure.

RATE CONTROL THERAPY

Multiple medications can be used for rate control therapy, with a general goal of maintaining a resting heart rate of 60 to 80 beats per minute (bpm) and heart rates during activity of 90 to 110 bpm.[2] Current guidelines recommend a less stringent approach based on the results of the RACE II trial in which lenient rate control (Heart rate control <110 bpm) was as effective as strict rate control (HR <80 bpm) in preventing cardiovascular events including heart failure hospitalizations, stroke, arrhythmias, and cardiovascular death.[6] Importantly, the RACE II trial excluded subjects with class IV heart failure or recent heart failure admissions and, therefore, response to rate control treatment may be different in those populations. Aggressive heart rate control and/or rhythm control is essential in situations in which elevated ventricular rates contribute to or cause ventricular dysfunction, an entity known as tachycardia-mediated cardiomyopathy. Medications most frequently used to achieve rate control include beta blockers, CCBs, and digoxin, which all assist in slowing AV node conduction. Beta blockers are potent AV nodal blockers and are effective in the acute setting because they have a rapid onset of action. In patients who are hemodynamically stable, β-blockers are effective medications for rate control but practitioners should use caution when using these medications in patients with hypotension or acutely exacerbated heart failure. Nondihydropyridine CCBs, including diltiazem and verapamil, can also be used in AF patients with preserved left ventricular systolic function. They are also more useful than beta blockers in patients with severe obstructive lung disease. CCBs have a relatively rapid onset of action and short half-life, and are frequently used as a continuous drip in hospitalized patients when a steady state of medication is most important. However, CCBs should not be used in patients with known left ventricular dysfunction because they are strong negative inotropes and their use may lead to worsening heart failure decompensation in those patients. Digoxin, which is a much weaker AV nodal blocker than either β-blockers or CCBs, was originally used in heart failure patients because it was shown to improve symptoms and quality of life. Recent evidence has, however, demonstrated that long-term use may actually increase the risk of death in the heart failure population.[7,8] Digoxin is most effective in hospitalized, bedbound patients, or those who will be mostly sedentary in an outpatient setting. It is much less effective when used in an active patient in the outpatient setting.

RHYTHM CONTROL
Restoring Sinus Rhythm

Rhythm control is a mainstay of therapy in patients with very symptomatic AF, either of new onset or of the recurrent persistent type. Restoration of sinus rhythm with DC cardioversion or pharmacologically is a reasonable goal in either of these patient populations. Importantly, the duration of AF must be taken into account because trials have shown low maintenance of sinus rhythm in subjects with long-standing arrhythmia.[9] Stroke prevention and anticoagulation are critical considerations in preparation for cardioversion given the high risk of thromboembolic events at the time of cardioversion and during the 3 to 4 weeks following the cardioversion. The risk has been shown to be as high as 5%.[10,11] If it can be clearly ascertained that the AF started 48 hours or less before presentation, trials have shown that the likelihood of thrombus formation is exceedingly low and, therefore, guidelines do not recommend routine anticoagulation before cardioversion.[1] For patients presenting with AF 48 hours or longer in duration, one can either initiate anticoagulation and continue it for at least 3 weeks before attempting cardioversion or perform a transesophageal echocardiogram–guided cardioversion, provided no thrombus is seen in the atrium. These 2 strategies were compared head to head in the Assessment of Cardioversion using Transesophageal Echocardiography trial, which revealed no difference between them in terms of embolic events or mortality. The trial was undertaken when only warfarin was available and it did find that hemorrhagic events were significantly lower and that patients had a shorter time to cardioversion in the transesophageal echocardiogram–guided cardioversion group.[12] The DC cardioversion itself uses short-acting sedation with external defibrillation pads placed in an anterior-posterior position across the chest wall. Energy selection is based on clinician preference, size of the patient, and duration of AF because higher levels of energy delivery are often required in patients with larger chests and longer duration of AF.[13,14] Cardioversion is commonly used in conjunction with antiarrhythmic medications to increase the likelihood of maintenance of sinus rhythm, especially in the long-standing persistent arrhythmia patients, or in those who have had frequent recurrent episodes of AF and have required multiple electrical cardioversions.

For infrequent symptomatic paroxysmal AF, class IC antiarrhythmic medications, including flecainide and propafenone, may be prescribed as needed with a so-called pill-in-the-pocket approach. This approach involves the self-administration of a single dose of flecainide (200–300 mg) or propafenone (450–600 mg) to restore sinus rhythm after the start of symptomatic palpitations. This treatment should include coadministration of an AV nodal blocking medication. Specifically, the patient should also take either a β-blocker or CCB approximately 30 minutes before administration of flecainide to prevent a rapid ventricular response if conversion to atrial flutter were to occur. When using this approach, the first dose should be administered under monitored conditions for safety considerations.[15] Another antiarrhythmic agent that is indicated for acute cardioversion of AF is ibutilide, which is an intravenous class III drug used in the emergency room for recent onset AF.[16]

Maintenance of Sinus Rhythm

DC cardioversion alone does not guarantee maintenance of sinus rhythm. In fact, up to 75% of patients will have a recurrence of AF within 1 year. AADs decrease the likelihood of recurrences. However, all of the available AADs have important side-effects and proarrhythmic potential. Appropriate AAD selection must take into account the drug's safety profile, the patient's clinical substrate, and the AF burden. The 2 drug classes that are most commonly used in the treatment of AF are class IC drugs, which block the sodium ion (Na^+) channel, and class III drugs, which are potent potassium ion (K^+) channel blockers.[16]

Class 1C drugs are contraindicated in patients who have structural heart disease, significant left ventricular hypertrophy, coronary artery disease, or congestive heart failure due to their proarrhythmic potential and negative inotropic properties.[16] The 2 most commonly used drugs in this class are flecainide and propafenone, which, in patients with structurally normal hearts, have relatively low risk of systemic side effects. The RAFT study (Rhythmol Atrial Fibrillation Trial) evaluated different doses of propafenone and found that the recurrence of AF in the propafenone group was significantly greater than or equal to in the placebo group. In terms of overall efficacy of the drug, propafenone significantly lengthened the time to first symptomatic atrial arrhythmia but there was also an increased incidence of adverse effects with increased doses of the drug (425 mg twice daily), leading to higher withdrawal rates.[17] The most common side effect of propafenone is nausea and vomiting, whereas flecainide can cause hair loss, tremors, visual disturbances, and headaches. Procainamide, an infrequently used class 1A AAD, is indicated, per guidelines, for use in hemodynamically stable patients with AF and Wolff-Parkinson-White syndrome.[18]

The 2 most frequently used class III AADs are dofetilide and sotalol. Sotalol (Betapace) is not only a K^+ channel blocker but also a nonselective β-blocker. In the SAFE-T study (Sotalol Amiodarone Atrial Fibrillation Efficacy Trial), sotalol was found to significantly reduce the rate of AF recurrence when compared with placebo. However, it increased the risk of QT prolongation and development of polymorphic ventricular tachycardia (torsades de pointes).[19] Importantly, sotalol is contraindicated in patients with systolic heart failure or significant left ventricular hypertrophy. Dofetilide (Tikosyn) is also a strong inhibitor of the K^+ channel, markedly prolonging repolarization and thereby decreasing AF recurrences. Although only dofetilide has a mandatory requirement by the US Food and Drug Administration, both drugs should be initiated on an in-patient telemetry unit and followed with serial electrocardiograms to assess for QT_c prolongation until steady state is achieved (5–6 doses). The Danish Investigations of Arrhythmia and Mortality on Dofetilide (DIAMOND)-AF trial showed that dofetilide was safe and increased the probability of obtaining and maintaining sinus rhythm in subjects with left ventricular dysfunction when compared with placebo (79% vs 42%). In addition, most patients who developed threatening QT_c prolongation and torsades de pointes did so within the first 3 days of use.[20] Based on that finding, guidelines recommend avoiding other QT_c-prolonging medications and/or p-glycoprotein inhibitors (ie, diltiazem, verapamil, amiodarone, erythromycin, and several antifungal medications), as well as a minimum of at least a 72-hour in-hospital monitoring period for patients initiating a class III AAD. This is an important consideration for primary care physicians taking care of patients on these drugs. Finally, both of these drugs are renally excreted and should be used with caution, if at all, in patients with renal insufficiency.

The most efficacious drug in preventing AF recurrences is amiodarone. When one looks at multiple studies comparing AADs to each other and to placebo, amiodarone is approximately 60% successful at maintaining sinus rhythm within a year compared with approximately 50% for other AADs and approximately 25% for placebo. Amiodarone is primarily a class III AAD, although it has properties of all IV classes, likely contributing to both its potent efficacy and to the myriad of side effects. Because of significant long-term toxicity, amiodarone is considered a second-line treatment, reserved for patients who have contraindications to or are unable to tolerate other antiarrhythmic agents. Among the numerous side effects are hepatic toxicity, peripheral neuropathy, tremors, visual disturbances, skin changes, nausea, thyroid dysfunction, and pulmonary toxicity.[21]

Finally, the most recently released AAD is dronedarone (Multaq). Designed as a less toxic form of amiodarone without an iodine moiety, dronedarone has an improved safety profile with less tissue accumulation, shorter half-life, and decreased systemic toxicity. The American-Australian-African Trial With Dronedarone in Patients With Atrial Fibrillation or Atrial Flutter for the Maintenance of Sinus Rhythm Trial (ADONIS) and Efficacy & Safety of Dronedarone Versus Amiodarone for the Maintenance of Sinus Rhythm in Patients With Atrial Fibrillation (DIONYSOS) trials showed that Dronedarone is more effective than placebo but less effective than amiodarone.[22,23] The ANDROMEDA trial revealed that subjects with systolic heart failure had a higher mortality with the drug.[24] The PALLAS trial found an increased mortality when dronedarone was used in persistent AF.[25] Dronedarone is the least potent AAD, with a narrow range of appropriate clinical use. It should not be used in patients with systolic heart failure and persistent AF. The AADs described in this section are detailed in **Table 2**. Recommended use of these agents, as well as catheter ablation, in the overall rhythm control management of AF is outlined in **Fig. 1**.

ABLATION THERAPY
Catheter Ablation

The main goal of catheter ablation for treatment of AF is to isolate the pulmonary veins (PVs) from the body of the left atrium. This approach is based on the finding that the electrical impulses that trigger AF originate at the connection of the veins with the left atrium, as first described in the landmark paper by Haissaguerre and colleagues.[26] In addition to the primary goal of PV isolation (PVI), a wide range of additional adjunctive strategies are used depending on the clinical milieu (left atrial substrate modification, superior vena cava, and/or coronary sinus ablation, linear lesion in right and left atrium, and ablation in areas of potential organization or rotors). The technical aspects of the procedure vary with different operators but generally start with the use of intracardiac echocardiogram, fluoroscopy, and a mapping software system to create a 3-dimensional model of the left atrium and PVs. Venous access is obtained in the femoral veins and electrophysiology catheters are guided into the heart under fluoroscopic guidance. Transseptal access is achieved with intracardiac ultrasound to introduce catheters into the left atrium. Ablation techniques have used numerous energy sources, most commonly radiofrequency energy, all with the endpoint goal of encircling and thereby electrically isolating the PVs.

As per the most current guidelines, the only indication for AF catheter ablation is in patients with symptomatic paroxysmal AF who are refractory or intolerant to at least 1 AAD.[27] Catheter ablation has become the treatment of choice for this patient cohort

Table 2
Classification of antiarrhythmic drugs

Drug	Mechanism of Action	Major Adverse Effects
Class I		
IA: Procainamide	Na$^+$ channel blockade, K$^+$ channel blockade, prolongs action potential duration	Sinus bradycardia, hypotension, nausea, QT$_c$ prolongation torsades de pointes (rare)
IC: Flecainide	Na$^+$ channel blockade, QRS widening, may prolong action potential duration	Sinus bradycardia, monomorphic ventricular tachycardia, increased AV nodal conduction, visual changes, hair loss, headache
IC: Propafenone	Na$^+$ channel blockade, may prolong action potential duration	Sinus bradycardia, nausea monomorphic ventricular tachycardia, increased AV conduction, gastrointestinal disturbances, dizziness
Class III		
Amiodarone	Na$^+$ and K$^+$ channel blockade, prolongs action potential duration, has β-blocker and CCB effects	Sinus bradycardia, hepatic toxicity, tremors, peripheral neuropathy, visual disturbances skin changes, nausea, thyroid dysfunction, pulmonary toxicity, QT$_c$ prolongation or torsades de pointes (rare)
Dofetilide or ibutilide	K$^+$ channel blockade (I$_{kr}$), marked prolongation of the action potential	Polymorphic VT (torsades de pointes), marked QT$_c$ prolongation
Sotalol	K$^+$ channel blockade (I$_{kr}$), β-blockade	Sinus bradycardia, polymorphic VT (torsades de pointes), QT$_c$ prolongation
Dronedarone	Na$^+$ and K$^+$ channel blockade, prolongs action potential duration, has β-blocker and CCB effects	Sinus bradycardia, QT$_c$ prolongation, gastrointestinal disturbances, rash

mainly based on the results of clinical trials such as THERMOCOOL-AF, STOP-AF, and MANTRA-AF. THERMOCOOL-AF, sought to investigate the utility of catheter ablation compared with AADs in symptomatic AF subjects. The study concluded that ablation was associated with lower AF recurrences at 9 months when compared with AADs (16% vs 66%).[28] The STOP-AF trial used a novel cryoballoon ablation technology in highly symptomatic AF subjects who failed at least 1 AAD. It found that 70% of the subjects treated with PVI were free from AF at 1 year, compared with just 7% of subjects who were treated with AAD.[29] The MANTRA-AF trial only randomized paroxysmal AF subjects to AADs versus catheter ablation as first-line treatment. It showed that there was no difference between the 2 groups in cumulative AF burden but did find that the burden was significantly less at 2 years in the ablation group.[30] Subjects with persistent AF have generally not been as well represented in catheter ablation studies. In 1 such trial, the SARA trial, subjects with persistent AF who were refractory to AADs had a lower AF burden with ablation than with AADs (44% vs 70%).[31]

There has been emerging interest in the utility of ablation in heart failure patients who are typically more symptomatic from their arrhythmia. Recent trials have shown better cardiovascular outcomes with ablation compared with AADs.[32] The largest of

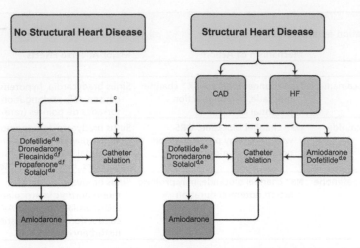

Fig. 1. Strategies for rhythm control in patients with paroxysmal[a] and persistent AF[b]. [a] Catheter ablation is only recommended as first-line therapy for patients with paroxysmal AF (class IIA recommendation). [b] Drugs are listed alphabetically. [c] Depending on patient preference when performed in experienced centers. [d] Not recommended with severe left ventricular hypertrophy (wall thickness >1.5 cm). [e] Should be used with caution in patients at risk for torsades de pointes ventricular tachycardia. [f] Should be combined with AV nodal blocking agents. CAD, coronary artery disease; HF, heart failure. (*From* January CT, Wann LS, Alpert JS, et al. 2014 AHA/ACC/HRS guideline for the management of patients with atrial fibrillation: a report of the American College of Cardiology/American Heart Association Task Force on Practice Guidelines and the Heart Rhythm Society. J Am Coll Cardiol 2014;64(21):e42; with permission.)

these trials, CASTLE-AF, randomized approximately 350 subjects to PVI ablation versus medical therapy (rate or rhythm control). After a median follow-up of approximately 40 months, ablation was associated with a 16% reduction in death or heart failure hospitalization. The reduction was driven by a nearly 12% absolute reduction in death between the 2 groups. Subjects randomized to ablation were also found to have an improvement in ejection fraction of 8% versus only 0.2% in the medical therapy group.[33] A recent meta-analysis of trials that studied ablation in heart failure patients showed that the results of CASTLE-AF aligned with the results of similar trials. Ablation resulted in lower mortality rates and heart failure hospitalizations. In addition, there were also improvements in ejection fraction, quality of life metrics, and functional capacity.[34]

Finally, the recent landmark CABANA trial studied more than 2000 subjects with AF and randomized subjects to PVI ablation versus drug therapy (rate or rhythm control). Results showed that ablation was not superior to drug therapy with respect to the primary endpoint of all-cause mortality, stroke, bleeding, or cardiac arrest. There was a significant reduction in the secondary endpoints of cardiovascular mortality or hospitalization, and a nearly 50% reduction in recurrent AF in the ablation group.[35]

Atrioventricular Nodal (AV Node) Ablation

For symptomatic AF patients who have exhausted every attempt at maintaining sinus rhythm, and in whom the ventricular rates remain uncontrolled despite the highest tolerated AV nodal blockers, it is reasonable to consider an AV nodal ablation.[36] This is really a permanent rate controlling strategy because the patient will remain in AF. It does obviate rate controlling medications but not the need for anticoagulation.

The procedure is fairly simple and brief, essentially creating complete AV block by scarring the tissue of the AV nodal junction. A single chamber ventricular pacemaker is needed to pace the ventricle, and the patient is made pacemaker-dependent. Some patients will develop left ventricular dysfunction from the chronic pacing, and controversy exists on whether patients with a normal left ventricular ejection fraction should receive a cardiac resynchronization device that paces the right and left ventricles simultaneously. Pacing from the His bundle may also prevent this long-term complication.

Surgical Ablation

Several surgical ablation techniques have been developed following the initial description of the Cox-Maze procedure by Dr James Cox and colleagues[37]. The original technique involved creating multiple scars using a cut-and-sew method throughout the left atrium to interrupt the signal propagation and prevent the triggers of AF. Currently, surgical ablation of AF is performed almost exclusively during concomitant open-heart procedures, such as bypass grafting or valve replacement. The modern Maze procedure has replaced the cut-and-sew method with surgical ablation tools that use radiofrequency or cryothermal energy to create the scar inside the left atrium.[38] Additionally, hybrid procedures have been developed with the goal of using both surgical epicardial ablation and endocardial PVI ablation. These newer techniques have shown promise in small trials but the long-term outcomes and efficacy are still being assessed.[39]

SUMMARY

Ultimately, the decision to follow a rate or rhythm control strategy has to take into account multiple factors, including patient symptoms and comorbidities, as well as physician and health system resources. As previously discussed, in patients with structurally normal hearts, rhythm control does not provide significant mortality benefit based on numerous large clinical trials.[40–42] Therefore, the focus should be placed on symptom control. In general, younger and more symptomatic patients tend to report greater improvement with rhythm control.[43] Moreover, clinicians often underestimate the true symptomatic burden of AF. In the authors' practices, most patients are treated with at least an initial attempt at restoring sinus rhythm. Many patients will experience a clear improvement in symptoms and overall energy level, even though they were thought to be asymptomatic before cardioversion. Importantly, one should recognize that rhythm control is often difficult, in particular with elderly patients, structurally abnormal hearts, valvular heart disease, potentially toxic AADs, and/or complications from ablation. Long-term rate versus rhythm control decisions should be shared between the physician and the patient with a clear discussion of the risks and benefits of attempted rhythm control versus rate control, with all of their respective limitations.

REFERENCES

1. Go AS, Hylek EM, Phillips KA, et al. Prevalence of diagnosed atrial fibrillation in adults: national implications for rhythm management and stroke prevention: the AnTicoagulation and Risk Factors in Atrial Fibrillation (ATRIA) Study. JAMA 2001;285(18):2370–5.

2. January C, Wann L, Alpert J, et al. 2014 AHA/ACC/HRS guideline for the management of patients with atrial fibrillation. J Am Coll Cardiol 2014;64(21):e1–76.

3. Kirchhof P, Benussi S, Kotecha D, et al. 2016 ESC guidelines for the management of atrial fibrillation developed in collaboration with EACTS. Eur Heart J 2016; 37(38):2893–962.

4. Atrial Fibrillation Follow-up Investigation of Rhythm Management (AFFIRM) Investigators. A comparison of rate control and rhythm control in patients with atrial fibrillation. N Engl J Med 2002;347(23):1825–33.

5. Van Gelder IC, Hagens VE, Bosker HA, et al. A comparison of rate control and rhythm control in patients with recurrent persistent atrial fibrillation. N Engl J Med 2002;347(23):1834–40.

6. Van Gelder IC, Groenveld HF, Crijns HJ, et al. Lenient versus strict rate control in patients with atrial fibrillation. N Engl J Med 2010;362(15):1363–73.

7. Digitalis Investigation Group. The effect of digoxin on mortality and morbidity in patients with heart failure. N Engl J Med 1997;336(8):525–33.

8. Vamos M, Erath JW, Hohnloser SH. Digoxin-associated mortality: a systematic review and meta-analysis of the literature. Eur Heart J 2015;36(28):1831–8.

9. Van Gelder IC, Crijns HJ, Van Gilst WH, et al. Prediction of uneventful cardioversion and maintenance of sinus rhythm from direct-current electrical cardioversion of chronic atrial fibrillation and flutter. Am J Cardiol 1991;68(1):41–6.

10. Hart RG, Benavente O, McBride R, et al. Antithrombotic therapy to prevent stroke in patients with atrial fibrillation: a meta-analysis. Ann Intern Med 1999;131(7): 492–501.

11. Bjerkelund CJ, Orning OM. The efficacy of anticoagulant therapy in preventing embolism related to DC electrical conversion of atrial fibrillation. Am J Cardiol 1969;23(2):208–16.

12. Klein AL, Grimm RA, Murray RD, et al. Use of transesophageal echocardiography to guide cardioversion in patients with atrial fibrillation. N Engl J Med 2001; 344(19):1411–20.

13. Kerber RE, Jensen SR, Grayzel J, et al. Elective cardioversion: influence of paddle-electrode location and size on success rates and energy requirements. N Engl J Med 1981;305(12):658–62.

14. Mittal S, Ayati S, Stein KM, et al. Transthoracic cardioversion of atrial fibrillation: comparison of rectilinear biphasic versus damped sine wave monophasic shocks. Circulation 2000;101(11):1282–7.

15. Alboni P, Botto GL, Baldi N, et al. Outpatient treatment of recent-onset atrial fibrillation with the "pill-in-the-pocket" approach. N Engl J Med 2004;351(23): 2384–91.

16. Lafuente-Lafuente C, Mouly S, Longás-Tejero MA, et al. Antiarrhythmic drugs for maintaining sinus rhythm after cardioversion of atrial fibrillation: a systematic review of randomized controlled trials. Arch Intern Med 2006;166(7):719–28.

17. Pritchett EL, Page RL, Carlson M, et al. Efficacy and safety of sustained-release propafenone (propafenone SR) for patients with atrial fibrillation. Am J Cardiol 2003;92(8):941–6.

18. Naccarelli GV, Wolbrette DL, Khan M, et al. Old and new antiarrhythmic drugs for converting and maintaining sinus rhythm in atrial fibrillation: comparative efficacy and results of trials. Am J Cardiol 2003;91(6):15–26.

19. Singh BN, Singh SN, Reda DJ, et al. Amiodarone versus sotalol for atrial fibrillation. N Engl J Med 2005;352(18):1861–72.

20. Pedersen OD, Bagger H, Keller N, et al. Efficacy of dofetilide in the treatment of atrial fibrillation-flutter in patients with reduced left ventricular function: a Danish investigations of arrhythmia and mortality on dofetilide (diamond) substudy. Circulation 2001;104(3):292–6.

21. Roy D, Talajic M, Dorian P, et al. Amiodarone to prevent recurrence of atrial fibrillation. N Engl J Med 2000;342(13):913–20.
22. Singh BN, Connolly SJ, Crijns HJ, et al. Dronedarone for maintenance of sinus rhythm in atrial fibrillation or flutter. N Engl J Med 2007;357(10):987–99.
23. Le Heuzey JY, De Ferrari GM, Radzik D, et al. A short-term, randomized, double-blind, parallel-group study to evaluate the efficacy and safety of dronedarone versus amiodarone in patients with persistent atrial fibrillation: the DIONYSOS study. J Cardiovasc Electrophysiol 2010;21(6):597–605.
24. Køber L, Torp-Pedersen C, McMurray JJ, et al. Increased mortality after dronedarone therapy for severe heart failure. N Engl J Med 2008;358(25):2678–87.
25. Connolly SJ, Camm AJ, Halperin JL, et al. Dronedarone in high-risk permanent atrial fibrillation. N Engl J Med 2011;365(24):2268–76.
26. Haissaguerre M, Jaïs P, Shah DC, et al. Spontaneous initiation of atrial fibrillation by ectopic beats originating in the pulmonary veins. N Engl J Med 1998;339(10):659–66.
27. Calkins H, Hindricks G, Cappato R, et al. 2017 HRS/EHRA/ECAS/APHRS/SOLAECE expert consensus statement on catheter and surgical ablation of atrial fibrillation. Europace 2017;20(1):e1–160.
28. Wilber DJ, Pappone C, Neuzil P, et al. Comparison of antiarrhythmic drug therapy and radiofrequency catheter ablation in patients with paroxysmal atrial fibrillation: a randomized controlled trial. JAMA 2010;303(4):333–40.
29. Packer DL, Kowal RC, Wheelan KR, et al. Cryoballoon ablation of pulmonary veins for paroxysmal atrial fibrillation: first results of the North American Arctic Front (STOP AF) pivotal trial. J Am Coll Cardiol 2013;61(16):1713–23.
30. Cosedis Nielsen J, Johannessen A, Raatikainen P, et al. Radiofrequency ablation as initial therapy in paroxysmal atrial fibrillation. N Engl J Med 2012;367(17):1587–95.
31. Mont L, Bisbal F, Hernandez-Madrid A, et al. Catheter ablation vs. antiarrhythmic drug treatment of persistent atrial fibrillation: a multicentre, randomized, controlled trial (SARA study). Eur Heart J 2013;35(8):501–7.
32. Di Biase L, Mohanty P, Mohanty S, et al. Ablation vs. amiodarone for treatment of persistent atrial fibrillation in patients with congestive heart failure and an implanted device: results from the AATAC multicenter randomized trial. Circulation 2016;133:1637–44.
33. Marrouche NF, Johannes B, Dietrich A, et al. Catheter ablation for atrial fibrillation with heart failure. N Engl J Med 2018;378(5):417–27.
34. Turagam MK, Garg J, Whang W, et al. Catheter ablation of atrial fibrillation in patients with heart failure: a meta-analysis of randomized controlled trials. Ann Intern Med 2019;170(1):41–50.
35. Packer DL, Mark DB, Robb RA, et al. Catheter ablation versus antiarrhythmic drug therapy for atrial fibrillation (CABANA) trial: study rationale and design. Am Heart J 2018;199:192–9.
36. Patel D, Daoud E. 2016 atrioventricular junction ablation for atrial fibrillation. Heart Fail Clin 2016;12(2):157–322.
37. Cox JL, Schuessler RB Jr, D'Agostino HJ, et al. The surgical treatment of atrial fibrillation. III. Development of a definitive surgical procedure. J Thorac Cardiovasc Surg 1991;101(4):569–83.
38. Ad N, Cox JL. The Maze procedure for the treatment of atrial fibrillation: a minimally invasive approach. J Card Surg 2004;19(3):196–200.

39. Gehi AK, Mounsey JP, Pursell I, et al. Hybrid epicardial-endocardial ablation using a pericardioscopic technique for the treatment of atrial fibrillation. Heart Rhythm 2013;10(1):22–8.
40. Hohnloser SH, Kuck KH, Lilienthal J. Rhythm or rate control in atrial fibrillation–Pharmacological Intervention in Atrial Fibrillation (PIAF): a randomised trial. Lancet 2000;356:1789.
41. Carlsson J, Miketic S, Windeler J, et al. Randomized trial of rate-control versus rhythm-control in persistent atrial fibrillation: the Strategies of Treatment of Atrial Fibrillation (STAF) study. J Am Coll Cardiol 2003;41:1690.
42. Guglin M, Chen R, Curtis AB. Sinus rhythm is associated with fewer heart failure symptoms: insights from the AFFIRM trial. Heart rhythm 2010;7(5):596–601.
43. Thrall G, Lane D, Carroll D, et al. Quality of life in patients with atrial fibrillation: a systematic review. Am J Med 2006;119(5):448.e1.

Stroke Prevention in Atrial Fibrillation
The Role of Oral Anticoagulation

Viwe Mtwesi, MB ChB, FCP(SA), Guy Amit, MD, MPH*

KEYWORDS

- Atrial fibrillation • Stroke prevention • Anticoagulation • NOAC • Warfarin

KEY POINTS

- Atrial fibrillation (AF) increases the risk of stroke by 5-fold, hence stroke prevention by anticoagulation is crucial for most patients.
- Novel oral anticoagulants are safer and more effective in most scenarios than warfarin for stroke prevention in nonvavlular AF.
- Subclinical AF, which is documented on rhythm monitoring and implantable devices, increases the risk of stroke. However, there are no clear guidelines for anticoagulation in this population of patients.

INTRODUCTION

Atrial fibrillation (AF) is the commonest arrhythmia seen on a day-to-day basis in clinical practice and is associated with increased risk of heart failure, stroke, and death.[1] It is an atrial tachyarrhythmia that is characterized by disorganized atrial electrical activity and results in atrial mechanical dysfunction. The diagnosis is usually made using an electrocardiogram showing no clear, consistent P waves but fibrillatory waves, which vary in size, shape, and timing and are associated with an irregular ventricular response.

At present, more than 33 million people have been documented to have AF worldwide and it is projected that, by 2050, in the united states alone AF prevalence will be 7.5 million.[2] Age seems to be an important risk for developing AF and its common cardioembolic complications. When AF occurs in the young, it is usually associated with structural heart conditions, or a strong genetic tendency. The prevalence escalates with increasing age[3] and men develop this arrhythmia more than women. It also seems

Disclosures: Dr G. Amit received honoraria from Pfizer, Bayer, and a research grant from Servier Canada.
Division of Cardiology, Department of Medicine, McMaster University, Hamilton General Hospital, 237 Barton Street East, Hamilton, Ontario L8L 2X2, Canada
* Corresponding author.
E-mail address: gamitmd@gmail.com

that race, and geographic distribution, tend to affect the prevalence of this condition. Epidemiologic studies have identified several risk factors for AF in addition to age and gender, of which the main ones are the presence of structural disease (mainly mitral valve disease), heart failure, hypertension, obesity, and sleep apnea (the Framingham study).[4]

AF causes a 4-fold to 5-fold increase in the risk of stroke, as established by the Framingham study,[5] and it also increases the risk of stroke independent of other risk factors for stroke. Roughly two-thirds of this stroke risk can be prevented with adequate oral anticoagulation.[6] Extensive work has been done regarding management of AF with special emphasis on preventing the most devastating outcome, stroke. Patients with AF tend to have bigger strokes and worse outcomes compared with other causes of stroke.[7] Patients with AF who are anticoagulated tend to have lower mortality and lower risks of developing ischemic stroke.[8,9] Although some clinical scenarios have clear management recommendations, many questions remain unanswered.

Clinical trials and guidelines have tried to address some of these gaps. Up until 2009, only antiplatelets and vitamin K antagonists were available for stroke prevention in AF. Unlike Aspirin (ASA), vitamin K antagonists have proven value. However, shortcomings include a narrow therapeutic index, significant food and drug interactions, and thus a need for constant monitoring. The benefits of warfarin are proportional to the time in therapeutic range (TTR).[10] The desired range is an International Normalized Ratio (INR) between 2.0 and 3.0.[11,12]

However, studies have shown TTR to be as low as 29% in patients with AF.[13] The low TTR is associated with both hemorrhagic events and strokes.[14,15]

Stroke prevention in AF involves weighing the risks and benefits of anticoagulation in the form of risk stratification. Once the diagnosis of AF is made, the risk of developing stroke must be assessed, as well as the bleeding risk on anticoagulation therapy. Risk stratification tools decrease morbidity and mortality.

Pathogenesis of Clot Formation

AF causes ineffective atrial contraction, blood stasis, and the risk of clot formation inside the left atrial appendage. There is a relationship between atrial appendage velocity and risk of stroke; low emptying flow rates of less than 250 mm/s have an increased incidence of stroke and peripheral embolic events.[16] AF promotes endothelial dysfunction and release of coagulation factors, namely thrombin and factor Xa. Endothelial dysfunction can cause the release of prothrombotic and proinflammatory molecules, including von Willebrand factor, selectins, and other vasoactive substances. C-reactive protein is a marker of inflammation and has been shown to have a direct relationship with stroke risk. Patients with the persistent form of AF have been shown to have higher levels of C-reactive protein compared with those in sinus rhythm.[17,18]

Classification of Atrial Fibrillation

Characterization of AF is important for the creation of a uniform nomenclature when describing patients, treatment, and clinical trials' populations. The American Heart Association (AHA) guidelines provide the following classification:

- Paroxysmal AF: AF that self-terminates intermittently or with intervention within 7 days of onset.
- Persistent AF: AF that fails to terminate within 7 days. Long-standing persistent AF is continuous and ongoing for greater than or equal to 12 months.

- Permanent AF: when a joint decision between patient and physician is made to no longer attempt restoration of sinus rhythm.
- Subclinical AF (SCAF): AF that is asymptomatic and found on monitoring devices or pacemakers. SCAF is currently defined by episodes that last greater than or equal to 30 seconds. However, the exact definition and the clinically important duration of SCAF remain controversial.
- Nonvalvular AF: AF in the absence of rheumatic mitral stenosis or a mechanical mitral prosthesis. Some cardiac societies extend this definition to the absence of any prosthetic heart valve and mitral valve repair.

RISK OF STROKE IN ATRIAL FIBRILLATION AND RISK STRATIFICATION
Types of Strokes, Prevalence of Atrial Fibrillation as the Cause of Stroke

Stroke risk increases by 5-fold in patients with AF.[19] Stroke associated with AF increases with age progressively, ranging from 6.7% in those aged 50 to 59 years to 36.2% in those aged 80 to 89 years.[5] In the United States about 100,000 to 125,000 embolic strokes per year are caused by AF, of which more than 20% are fatal. To be precise, 1 in 6 patients with stroke have AF as a cause, and 1 in 4 of the estimated 12 million ischemic strokes annually have no cause.[20,21] About 30% of patients with embolic stroke of undetermined source, which was previously referred to as cryptogenic stroke, are found to have paroxysmal AF on follow-up.[22] Whether the type of AF affects the risk of stroke is controversial. Paroxysmal AF was thought to confer the same stroke risk as chronic AF,[23] and this was substantiated with data from the ACTIVE-W study showing that incidence of stroke in paroxysmal versus sustained AF in patients taking oral anticoagulation or combined antiplatelet therapy is similar.[24] However, combined data from the aspirin arms of ACTIVE-A and AVERROES studies showed a yearly risk of ischemic stroke of 2.1%, 3.0%, and 4.2% for patients with paroxysmal, persistent, and permanent AF respectively. This difference in risk stayed significant after adjustment for comorbidities.[25] Most strokes in patients with AF are ischemic; the remainder that are hemorrhagic have an unclear cause because only a small fraction are caused by anticoagulation.[26]

Risk Stratification for Stroke in Atrial Fibrillation

The risk of stroke is different among patients with AF and the benefit of anticoagulation depends on that risk. Hence, prediction models are important to determine the clinical value and cost-effectiveness of thromboprophylaxis. Prediction models classify patients into low, moderate, and high risk.

The $CHADS_2$ (congestive heart failure, hypertension, age, diabetes, prior stroke) score is the most commonly used and the most validated. This stroke risk model has been shown to be accurate in prediction of stroke and selection of antithrombotic therapy.[27] The annual risk varies from 1.9% in $CHADS_2 = 0\%$ to 12.5% ($CHADS_2 = 6$). Like any risk stratification model, it has some shortfalls because it excludes some risk factors that are thought to be important in stroke prevention.[28]

The European Society of Cardiology has endorsed the use of the $CHAD_2DS_2$-VASc score to complement the $CHADS_2$ score.[29] This endorsement was based on registry data showing improvement in predictive value when CHA_2DS_2-VASc was used compared with $CHADS_2$.[30] The SPORTIF trial also showed a better prediction for the CHA_2DS_2-VASc, mainly providing a finer resolution at the lower risk end.[31] The ATRIA stroke risk score combines clinical factors with assessment of kidney function and was shown to perform better in identifying low-risk patients in a UK study compared with the scores discussed earlier. However, the need for blood and urine

Table 1 The different stroke risk scores in atrial fibrillation		
Risk Score	Score Range Risk of Stroke/Year (%)	Risk Score Range (Stroke Risk from Low to High)
CHADS$_2$[27]	0–6	1.9% – >8.5%
CHA$_2$DS$_2$-VaSc[29]	0–9	0.2% – 17.4%
ATRIA[32]	0–15	<1% – >2%

Abbreviations: ATRIA, age, female, diabetes, congestive heart failure, hypertension, proteinuria, estimated glomerular filtration rate less than 45 mL/min/1.73 m^2/end-stage renal disease; CHADS$_2$, cardiomyopathy/congestive heart failure, hypertension, age greater than 75 years, diabetes, stroke (2 points); CHA$_2$DS$_2$.VASc, cardiomyopathy/congestive heart failure, hypertension, age greater than 65 years/age greater than 75 years (2 points), diabetes, stroke (2 points), vascular disease, sex category (1 point for women).

tests make it less clinician friendly.[32] A comparison between the 3 main risk scores in shown in **Table 1**.

STROKE PREVENTION IN ATRIAL FIBRILLATION: ASPIRIN AND VITAMIN K ANTAGONISTS

The prevention of stroke is now the cornerstone of AF management.[33] A study by Hart and colleagues[34] found a temporal trend showing a decrease in AF-associated stroke incidence, likely because of wide use of antithrombotic therapy. This finding suggests that most AF-related strokes can be prevented by the use of oral anticoagulants.[35]

Table 2 is a summary of recommendations for anticoagulation according to the different guidelines.

Antiplatelet Agents

Aspirin has been the most studied. Hart and colleagues[34] combined 7 aspirin trials (aspirin vs placebo or vs no treatment) in a meta-analysis comprising 3990 patients with both primary and secondary prevention indications. Aspirin dosages ranged from 50 to 1200 mg/d. The relative risk reduction was 19% (95% confidence interval [CI], 1%–35%) suggesting no significant reduction. The combination of clopidogrel (Plavix) and aspirin resulted in a 28% relative risk reduction (95% CI, 17%–38%) in all strokes compared with aspirin alone.[36]

Table 2 Comparison between the different guidelines in respect to initiation of anticoagulation		
AHA/ACC/HRS 2019[81]	European Society of Cardiology 2016[18]	Canadian Cardiovascular Society 2018[70]
CHA$_2$DS$_2$-VASC = 0 No OAC	CHA$_2$DS$_2$-VASC = 0 No OAC	CHADS$_2$ = 0 No OAC
CHA$_2$DS$_2$-VASC = 1 Aspirin may be considered CHA$_2$DS$_2$-VASC ≥2 OAC	CHA$_2$DS$_2$-VASC ≥1 OAC	Age>65 y or CHADS$_2$ ≥1 OAC

Abbreviations: ACC, American College of Cardiology; HRS, Heart Rhythm Society; OAC, oral anticoagulant.

Warfarin

For decades, warfarin was the cornerstone for stroke prevention. A meta-analysis of 6 trials compared adjusted-dose warfarin with placebo and included 2900 patients. The stroke rate was 4.5%/y for primary prevention and 12%/y for secondary prevention among patients assigned to the placebo or control groups. The analysis showed a relative risk reduction of 64% (95% CI, 49%–74%).[35] Eleven trials compared adjusted-dose warfarin with antiplatelet therapy in more than 11,000 patients[35] Warfarin was associated with a 37% (CI, 23%–48%) reduction in strokes. The largest trial[37] studied 6706 and compared adjusted-dose warfarin with a combination of clopidogrel plus aspirin. Warfarin was associated with a relative risk reduction of 40% (CI, 18%–56%). The SPAF III study compared a combination of fixed-dose warfarin and aspirin with adjusted-dose warfarin in 1044 patients and showed again a clear superiority of the latter.[12] As discussed earlier, low TTR is associated with both stroke and bleeding.[14,15]

Studies have shown that there is still suboptimal use of anticoagulants and, for patients on warfarin, optimal control is a serious concern because, in some studies, up to 50% of patients do not reach acceptable ranges of INR.[38,39]

STROKE PREVENTION IN ATRIAL FIBRILLATION: NOVEL ORAL ANTICOAGULATION AGENTS

As a group, novel oral anticoagulants (NOACs) or direct oral anticoagulants are easier to use than warfarin, because they are administered in a fixed dose without need for monitoring. Their mechanism of action is different, as well as their pharmacokinetics and pharmacodynamics.

Fig. 1 shows the clotting cascade and the mechanism of action of the different NOACs, and **Table 3** shows their properties and the major trial data.

Dabigatran Etexilate (Pradaxa)

Dabigatran etexilate (Pradaxa) is a direct thrombin inhibitor with a half-life of 12 to 17 hours. Eighty percent of the dose of the drug is excreted by the kidneys.[40] Dabigatran use in nonvalvular AF was studied in the RE-LY (Randomized Evaluation of Long-

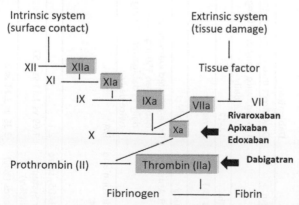

Fig. 1. Mechanism of action of NOACs. (*Adapted from* Meka YH, Mekaj AY, Duci SB, et al. New oral anticoagulants: their advantages and disadvantages compared with vitamin K antagonists in the prevention and treatment of patients with thromboembolic events. Ther Clin Risk Manag 2015;11:969.)

Table 3
The major novel oral anticoagulant properties and trials

	Dabigatran	Rivaroxaban	Apixaban	Edoxaban
Mechanism	Oral direct thrombin inhibitor	Oral direct factor Xa inhibitor	Oral direct factor Xa inhibitor	Oral direct factor Xa inhibitor
Dosing	150 mg twice daily or 110 mg twice daily	20 mg once daily	5 mg twice daily	60 mg once daily or 30 mg once daily
Half-life (h)	12–17	5–13	9–14	10–14
Excretion (%)	80 renal	66 liver 33 renal	27 renal	50 renal
Major Study	RE-LY[58]	ROCKET-AF[59]	ARISTOTLE[42]	ENGAGE AF-TIMI 48[45]
Treatment Arms	Dose-adjusted warfarin vs dabigatran 150 mg twice daily vs dabigatran 110 mg twice daily	Dose-adjusted warfarin vs rivaroxaban 20 mg once daily	Dose-adjusted warfarin vs apixaban 5 mg twice daily	Dose-adjusted warfarin vs edoxaban 60 mg once daily vs edoxaban 30 mg once daily
Dose Reduction and Criteria	NA	15 mg once daily CrCl 30–49 mL/min	2.5 mg twice daily if 2 out of 3 of the following: age >80 y, weight <60 kg, or creatinine >133 mmol/L	Dose halved if CrCl 30–50 mL/min, weight ≤60 kg, or concomitant use of verapamil or quinidine
Mean CHADS$_2$ score	2.1	3.5	2.1	2.8
Stroke or Systemic Emboli (%/y)	1.69 vs 1.11 vs 1.53	2.20 vs 1.70	1.60 vs 1.27	1.50 vs 1.18 vs 1.61
Major Bleeds (%/y)	3.36 vs 3.11 vs 2.71	3.40 vs 3.60	3.09 vs 2.13	3.43 vs 2.75 vs 1.61

Abbreviations: CrCl, creatinine clearance; NA, not available.

Term Anticoagulation Therapy) trial, an open-label randomized comparison of dabigatran (110 mg or 150 mg twice daily) with adjusted-dose warfarin over 2 years in 18,113 patients with nonvalvular AF. Patients with creatinine clearance less than or equal to 30 mL/min were excluded. The primary outcome was stroke or systemic embolism. This outcome occurred in 1.53%, 1.11%, and 1.69% of patients in the 110-mg dabigatran, 150-mg dabigatran, and warfarin groups, respectively. Dabigatran 150 mg significantly reduced strokes compared with warfarin with similar risk of major bleeding, whereas dabigatran 110 mg had a similar rate of stroke as warfarin with significantly reduced major bleeding. Both doses markedly reduced intracerebral, life-threatening, and total bleeding risk with 0.38% yearly rate of hemorrhagic stroke on warfarin compared with 0.12% in the 110-mg dabigatran and 0.10% in the 150-mg group. The net clinical benefit outcome (vascular events, death, and major bleed) favored 150-mg dabigatran rather than warfarin. In the United States, the Food and Drug Administration (FDA) also approved PRADAXA 75 mg twice daily for patients who have severe renal impairment.

Rivaroxaban (Xarelto)

Rivaroxaban (Xarelto) is a direct factor Xa inhibitor, mainly excreted by the kidneys, with a small fraction metabolized by the liver. It is administered in a single daily evening dose with food. Rivaroxaban was studied in the ROCKET AF (Rivaroxaban Once Daily Oral Direct Factor Xa Inhibition Compared with Vitamin K Antagonism for Prevention of Stroke and Embolism Trial in Atrial Fibrillation), which was a double-blind study of 14,264 patients with nonvalvular AF with a mean age of 73 years and a mean follow-up of more than 2 years. The study compared a 20-mg dose (15 mg if the creatinine clearance was <50 mL/min) with warfarin. Subjects with a creatinine clearance of less than 30 mL/min were excluded. Patients in ROCKET AF were older and had a greater mean $CHADS_2$ score of 3.4 than in the RE-LY Trial. The primary end point was stroke or systemic embolism, which occurred in 1.7%/y versus 2.2%/y in the rivaroxaban and warfarin groups, respectively, showing noninferiority. Any bleeding occurred at a rate of 14.9%/y with rivaroxaban versus 14.5%/y with warfarin. There were significantly fewer intracranial hemorrhages (0.5% vs 0.7%; $P = .02$) and fatal bleedings (0.2% vs 0.5%; $P = .003$) in the rivaroxaban compared with the warfarin group.

Apixaban (Eliquis)

Apixaban (Eliquis) is a direct factor Xa inhibitor predominantly excreted by the liver, with a half-life of 12 hours.[41] Apixaban was tested in the ARISTOTLE (Apixaban Versus Warfarin in Patients with Atrial Fibrillation) a double-blind randomized trial with 18,201 patients with nonvalvular AF followed for 1.8 years. Apixaban 5 mg twice daily was compared with warfarin. The dose of apixaban was adjusted in patients with 2 out of 3 of the following: age greater than 80 years, weight less than 60 kg, or creatinine greater than 133 mmol/L. The primary outcome was stroke and systemic embolism. It occurred at a rate of 1.27%/y in the apixaban group and 1.60%/y in the warfarin group ($P<.001$ for noninferiority and $P = .01$ for superiority). The major bleeding rate was also significantly lower in the apixaban group at 2.13%/y compared with 3.09%/y in the warfarin group. The hemorrhagic stroke rate was 0.24%/y versus 0.47%/y in the warfarin group. Apixaban was also studied versus aspirin in the AVERROES study, which was a double-blind study of 599 patients with a $CHADS_2$ score of 2. This study was stopped prematurely because of superiority of apixaban in preventing stroke, with a risk reduction of 55% compared with aspirin. Bleeding risk was similar between the 2 groups.[42] In both studies, patients with creatinine clearance less than 25 mL/min were excluded. However, there are data to support the use of apixaban in patients on hemodialysis, as discussed later.[43]

Edoxaban (Savaysa)

Edoxaban (Savaysa) is a direct factor Xa inhibitor with a half-life between 10 and 14 hours and with 50% kidney excretion. This drug was tested in the ENGAGE AF-TIMI (Effective Anticoagulation with Factor Xa Next Generation in Atrial Fibrillation–Thrombolysis in Myocardial Infarction) trial.[44] High-dose edoxaban (60 mg once daily) and low-dose edoxaban (30 mg once daily) were compared with warfarin. The drug dose was halved if any of the following were present: estimated creatinine clearance of 30 to 50 mL/min, weight less than or equal to 60 kg, or the concomitant use of verapamil or quinidine.[45] The higher dose of edoxaban reduced the primary end point of stroke or systemic embolism by 21% (1.18%/y vs 1.50%/y) and bleeding risk by 20% (2.75%/y vs 3.43%/y) compared with warfarin. The low dose was noninferior to warfarin for stroke prevention and, notably, reduced bleeding risk by 53%. The rate of death was lower for both 60-mg and 30-mg doses. In spite of the impressive bleeding reduction with the 30-mg dose, only the 60-mg dose is approved for stroke prevention.[44]

MONITORING AND REVERSAL OF NOVEL ORAL ANTICOAGULANTS

The predictable anticoagulant effect of NOACs has provided the pharmacologic basis for administration in fixed doses without routine laboratory monitoring.[46] A meta-analysis by Ruff and colleagues[6] showed that fixed-dose NOAC therapy is associated with less bleeding and has the same efficacy as dose-adjusted warfarin. Dabigatran monitoring is assessed by diluted thrombin clotting time and ecarin-based essay, and these have a linear relationship with dabigatran concentration.[47] Monitoring of apixaban, edoxaban, and rivaroxaban is done by chromogenic anti–factor Xa,[48] and absence of anti–factor Xa activity indicates the absence of these drugs in the system.[49] The biggest problem with these assays is that they are not freely available and turnaround time is slow.[50]

Drug reversal is often needed when patients have life-threatening bleeding while on NOACs. For dabigatran, idarucizumab has been proved effective as a reversal agent. It is a humanized monoclonal antibody fragment that binds to free and thrombin-bound dabigatran within minutes of administration.[51] The REVERSE AD study investigated the safety and efficacy of 5 g of idarucizumab in 503 patients on dabigatran who received idarucizumab for either active bleeding or preprocedure reversal. Of the 203 evaluable patients treated for bleeding, 68% had cessation of bleeding within 24 hours. In the 197 patients who had surgery, hemostasis was reported to be normal in 93%.[52]

Similar agents for factor Xa inhibitors are under development, such as andexanet alfa (a recombinant human factor Xa analogue that competes for the factor Xa receptors with factor Xa inhibitors) and aripazine, a small synthetic molecule that seems to have more generalized antagonistic effects. Andexanet was approved by the FDA in May of 2018 for the reversal of anticoagulation in patients with life-threatening bleeding taking rivaroxaban and apixaban. It is a modified human recombinant factor Xa decoy protein. The preliminary report from the ANNEXA-4 study provided evidence for efficacy of andexanet in 47 patients with bleeding who were on factor Xa drugs.[53] More studies are currently underway to further investigate this reversal agent.

In cases of severe bleeding, when idarucizumab is not readily available, or in case bleeding occurs in patients treated with any of the factor Xa inhibitors, clinicians can resort to nonspecific reversal strategies. Some studies have confirmed the effects of prothrombin complex concentrate (PCC) or activated prothrombin complex concentrate (aPCC). However, the efficacy of PCC or aPCC in patients who are actively bleeding has not been firmly established, and the potential prothrombotic effects should always be a concern.[54]

STROKE PREVENTION IN VALVULAR ATRIAL FIBRILLATION

Valvular AF refers to AF that occurs in patients with either significant (moderate to severe) rheumatic mitral stenosis or mechanical heart valves.[18] The AHA includes patients with mitral valve repair in their definition of valvular AF.[55] Because there is no consensus, De Caterina and Camm[56] coined the term mechanical and rheumatic mitral valvular AF. Valvular disease is associated with a 1.8-fold to 3.4-fold increase in risk of AF.[57] Moreover, most of the trials discussed earlier excluded patients with valvular AF. Note that in the nonvalvular AF trials, the definition of valvular AF varied. Thus, RE-LY excluded patients who had a prosthetic valve or significant left-sided valve disease.[58] In contrast, ROCKET AF only excluded patients with significant mitral valve disease and prosthetic heart valves, and included patients with annuloplasty or valvuloplasty.[59] In ARISTOTLE, 26% of patients had at least moderate to severe valve disease. Such patients were found to have the same stroke reduction and major bleeding benefits. The same criteria were used in the ENGAGE-AF trial.[44]

The RE-ALIGN study compared dabigatran with warfarin for prevention of thromboembolism in patients with mechanical heart valves (mitral or aortic). The study was terminated early because of an excess of both ischemic stroke and bleeding in the dabigatran group. Specifically, ischemic or unspecified stroke occurred in 5% of the dabigatran group but in none of the patients in the warfarin group.[60] The results of this study prompted a black box warning against the use of dabigatran or other NOACs in patients with mechanical heart valves. Therefore, patients with AF with mechanical heart valves need to be treated with warfarin or another vitamin K antagonist.

Although NOACs are contraindicated in patients with mechanical valves, limited data are available regarding patients with bioprosthetic valves. In these patients, it is customary to use warfarin for the first 3 to 6 months after valve replacement, but there is no need for chronic anticoagulation, and aspirin is usually prescribed. A small echocardiographic study showed no difference in the rate of intracardiac thrombus or embolic events between dabigatran and warfarin[61] in patients with bioprosthetic valves. A retrospective subanalysis of 82 patients from ARISTOTLE also found no difference in stroke/systemic embolism (2.9% with apixaban vs 0% with warfarin; P value not significant).[62] A retrospective analysis of 191 patients with bioprosthetic valves from ENGAGE AF found that the rates of stroke/systemic embolism were similar for high-dose and low-dose edoxaban versus warfarin.

The INVICTUS-VKA trial (Investigation of rheumatic AF Treatment Using Vitamin K Antagonists or Rivaroxaban) is an ongoing prospective randomized noninferiority trial testing the hypothesis that rivaroxaban is noninferior to warfarin in preventing stoke or systemic embolism in patients with rheumatic valvular AF.[63]

STROKE PREVENTION IN ATRIAL FIBRILLATION AND RENAL DYSFUNCTION

Patients with chronic kidney disease (CKD) are another group at a higher risk of stroke because AF is common in these individuals.[64] The prevalence of AF in dialysis patients is between 8% and 34% (7% for peritoneal dialysis), which is double the prevalence of patients without renal disease.[65] in patients with advanced CKD has been of concern, but NOACs have been found to have equal safety, and possibly greater efficacy, compared with warfarin.[53,58,59] Patients with a creatinine clearance of less than or equal to 30 mL/min pose a difficult clinical dilemma, because most of these patients were excluded from clinical trials.

Recently, pharmacologic data showed that, in patients on dialysis, apixaban 2.5 mg twice daily resulted in a steady-state drug exposure comparable with that of 5 mg twice daily in patients with preserved renal function.[63] A recent trial compared apixaban (5 mg vs 2.5 mg twice daily) and warfarin in dialysis patients. Standard-dose apixaban was associated with a lower risk of death than that observed with low-dose apixaban and warfarin, and there was a lower risk of major bleeding with apixaban than with warfarin.[66] The current AHA/American College of Cardiology (ACC)/Heart Rhythm Society (HRS) guideline states that "for patients with AF who have a CHA_2DS_2-VASc score of ≥ 2 (men) or ≥ 3 (women) and who have end-stage chronic kidney disease (CKD; creatinine clearance [CrCl] <15 mL/min) or are on dialysis, it might be reasonable to prescribe warfarin (INR 2.0–3.0) or apixaban for oral anticoagulation."[67]

STROKE PREVENTION IN SUBCLINICAL ATRIAL FIBRILLATION

In the era of pacemakers, implantable defibrillators, and long-term monitoring devices, many AF episodes that are asymptomatic are being captured via the device memories. At present there is no consensus regarding SCAF in terms of the length of a qualifying episode, or for whether SCAF is an indication for anticoagulation therapy. In the ASSERT trial, 2580 patients greater than or equal to 65 years old with an implanted pacemaker or defibrillator and no history of AF were monitored for 3 months to detect SCAF (defined as episodes with an atrial rate >190 beats/min for ≥ 6 minutes). At 3 months the rate of SCAF was 10%. Over a mean follow-up of 2.5 years, SCAF episodes were associated with an increased risk of clinical AF (hazard ratio, 5.6) and of ischemic stroke or systemic embolism (hazard ratio, 2.5).[68] The TRENDS study, of similar design, correlated the burden of SCAF with the risk of stroke and showed that SCAF of greater than 5.5 hours doubled the risk of stroke.[69] Although SCAF is associated with stroke, this risk seems to be low compared with the stroke risk in patients with similar risk profiles and clinical AF.[61,62] Given the uncertainty of the risk/benefit ratio of oral anticoagulation for stroke prevention in patients with device-detected SCAF, specific recommendations in most guidelines for AF management are scarce. The 2014 Canadian Cardiovascular Society Guidelines recommend oral anticoagulation therapy for patients with SCAF who are greater than or equal to 65 years old, with a $CHADS_2$ greater than or equal to 1 and episodes that last more than 24 hours, or for shorter episodes only if the patient is high risk, such as having a history of recent cryptogenic stroke.[70] Although the new AHA/ACC/HRS AF guidelines acknowledge the need to monitor for SCAF especially in patients after a cryptogenic stroke, they provide no recommendation for when treatment is necessary.[71] The ongoing Apixaban for the Reduction of Thrombo-Embolism in Patients With Device-Detected Sub-Clinical Atrial Fibrillation (ARTESiA) trial is comparing apixaban with aspirin in a double-blind manner in patients with SCAF greater than or equal to 6 minutes but less than 24 hours and moderate to high risk of stroke.[72]

STROKE PREVENTION AROUND CARDIOVERSION

After cardioversion (electrical or pharmacologic) the atrial mechanical function (contraction of the left atrial appendage) can take several weeks to recover, which makes anticoagulation critical during this period of time.[73] It is well documented that embolic events are increased around the time of cardioversion,[74,75] with the peak being 10 days after reversion to sinus rhythm.[76,77] The risk of embolic events increases by more than 60% in patients with AF longer than 48 hours and not treated with anticoagulants after cardioversion.[58,73,78] Patients that have AF for greater than 48 hours and no urgent indication for cardioversion should therefore be placed on anticoagulation for at least 3 weeks before they are cardioverted.[79] The use of transesophageal echocardiography to exclude left atrial appendage clot can be an alternative to precardioversion anticoagulation. Although the risk of embolization is low in acute AF of less than or equal to 48 hours' duration, the risk is not negligible. A recent Finnish study found that the risk of stroke after cardioversion in patients with AF less than or equal to 48 hours correlated with their $CHADS_2$ score.[80] There was also a significantly lower risk in patients with AF of less than or equal to 12 hours in duration.[80] Following these data, the new Canadian AF guidelines recommend that only patients with nonvalvular AF of less than 12 hours, or patients with AF of less than 48 hours with $CHADS_2$ score less than 2, can be safely cardioverted without prior anticoagulation or transesophageal echo.[81] The 2019 update to the ACC/AHA/HRS AF guidelines recommends that it is reasonable to give heparin, a factor Xa inhibitor, or a direct thrombin inhibitor as soon as possible before cardioversion, followed by long-term anticoagulation therapy for patients with AF of less than or equal to 48 hours' duration and with a CHA_2DS_2-VASc greater than or equal to 2 in men and greater than or equal to 3 in women.[81]

NOACs have shown equal, if not better, outcomes compared with warfarin in the pericardioversion period. X-VeRT was the first prospective trial for NOAC use before cardioversion; it randomized 1504 patients to rivaroxaban versus dose-adjusted warfarin. The primary efficacy outcome (a composite of stroke, transient ischemic attack, systemic embolism, myocardial infarction, and cardiovascular death) occurred in 0.51% of the rivaroxaban group and 1.02% of the warfarin group.[82] The EMANATE (Eliquis Evaluated in Acute Cardioversion Compared to Usual Treatments for Anticoagulation in Subjects with AF) trial suggested a rapid loading regimen for apixaban in patients in need for acute cardioversion.[83] It required greater than or equal to 5 doses of apixaban or a single 10-mg loading dose, after which a cardioversion could be performed 2 hours after the load or in the usual manner. The trial randomized 1500 patients to apixaban or heparin/warfarin before and after cardioversion. Of the patients who did not undergo transesophageal echocardiography, cardioversion was performed faster in the apixaban group (median of 1 day for the rapid loading group, 30 days for the usual loading group, and 43 days for the heparin/warfarin group). There was a clear benefit to apixaban in the primary end point of stroke or systemic embolism at 30 days after cardioversion (0% vs 0.8%).[83]

REFERENCES

1. Hylek EM, Go AS, Chang Y, et al. Effect of intensity of oral anticoagulation on stroke severity and mortality in atrial fibrillation. N Engl J Med 2003;349(11): 1019–26.

2. Naccarelli GV, Varker H, Lin J, et al. Increasing prevalence of atrial fibrillation and flutter in the United States. Am J Cardiol 2009;104(11):1534–9.

3. Go AS, Hylek EM, Phillips KA, et al. Prevalence of diagnosed atrial fibrillation in adults: national implications for rhythm management and stroke prevention: the AnTicoagulation and Risk Factors in Atrial Fibrillation (ATRIA) Study. JAMA 2001;285(18):2370–5.

4. Schnabel RB, Sullivan LM, Levy D, et al. Development of a risk score for atrial fibrillation (Framingham Heart Study): a community-based cohort study. Lancet 2009;373(9665):739–45.
5. Wolf PA, Abbott RD, Kannel WB. Atrial fibrillation: a major contributor to stroke in the elderly. The Framingham Study. Arch Intern Med 1987;147(9):1561–4.
6. Ruff CT, Giugliano RP, Braunwald E, et al. Comparison of the efficacy and safety of new oral anticoagulants with warfarin in patients with atrial fibrillation: a meta-analysis of randomised trials. Lancet 2014;383(9921):955–62.
7. Miller PSJ, Andersson FL, Kalra L. Are cost benefits of anticoagulation for stroke prevention in atrial fibrillation underestimated? Stroke 2005;36(2):360–6.
8. Marini C, De Santis F, Sacco S, et al. Contribution of atrial fibrillation to incidence and outcome of ischemic stroke: results from a population-based study. Stroke 2005;36(6):1115–9.
9. Jørgensen HS, Nakayama H, Jakob R, et al. Acute stroke with atrial fibrillation. Stroke 1996;27(10):1765–9.
10. Connolly SJ, Pogue J, Eikelboom J, et al. Benefit of oral anticoagulant over anti-platelet therapy in atrial fibrillation depends on the quality of international normalized ratio control achieved by centers and countries as measured by time in therapeutic range. Circulation 2008;118(20):2029–37.
11. Albers GW, Diener H-C, Frison L, et al. Ximelagatran vs warfarin for stroke prevention in patients with nonvalvular atrial fibrillation: a randomized trial. JAMA 2005;293(6):690–8.
12. Blackshear J, Baker V, Rubino F, et al. Adjusted-dose warfarin versus low-intensity, fixed-dose warfarin plus aspirin for high-risk patients with atrial fibrillation: Stroke Prevention in Atrial Fibrillation III randomised clinical trial. Lancet 1996;348(9028):633–8.
13. Samsa GP, Matchar DB, Goldstein LB, et al. Quality of anticoagulation management among patients with atrial fibrillation: results of a review of medical records from 2 communities. Arch Intern Med 2000;160(7):967–73.
14. White HD, Gruber M, Feyzi J, et al. Comparison of outcomes among patients randomized to warfarin therapy according to anticoagulant control: results from SPORTIF III and V. Arch Intern Med 2007;167(3):239–45.
15. Pokorney SD, Simon DN, Thomas L, et al. Patients' time in therapeutic range on warfarin among US patients with atrial fibrillation: results from ORBIT-AF registry. Am Heart J 2015;170(1):141–8, 148.e1.
16. Kim Y-H, Roh S-Y. The mechanism of and preventive therapy for stroke in patients with atrial fibrillation. J Stroke 2016;18(2):129–37.
17. Watson T, Shantsila E, Lip GYH. Mechanisms of thrombogenesis in atrial fibrillation: Virchow's triad revisited. Lancet 2009;373(9658):155–66.
18. Kirchhof P, Benussi S, Kotecha D, et al. 2016 ESC guidelines for the management of atrial fibrillation developed in collaboration with EACTS. Eur Heart J 2016; 37(38):2893–962.
19. Wolf PA, Abbott RD, Kannel WB. Atrial fibrillation as an independent risk factor for stroke: the Framingham Study. Stroke 1991;22(8):983–8.
20. Bal S, Patel SK, Almekhlafi M, et al. High rate of magnetic resonance imaging stroke recurrence in cryptogenic transient ischemic attack and minor stroke patients. Stroke 2012;43(12):3387–8.
21. Hart RG, Diener H-C, Coutts SB, et al. Embolic strokes of undetermined source: the case for a new clinical construct. Lancet Neurol 2014;13(4):429–38.
22. Petty GW, Brown RD, Whisnant JP, et al. Ischemic stroke subtypes: a population-based study of incidence and risk factors. Stroke 1999;30(12):2513–6.

23. Hart RG, Pearce LA, Rothbart RM, et al. Stroke with intermittent atrial fibrillation: incidence and predictors during aspirin therapy. Stroke Prevention in Atrial Fibrillation Investigators. J Am Coll Cardiol 2000;35(1):183–7.
24. Hohnloser SH, Pajitnev D, Pogue J, et al. Incidence of stroke in paroxysmal versus sustained atrial fibrillation in patients taking oral anticoagulation or combined antiplatelet therapy: an ACTIVE W Substudy. J Am Coll Cardiol 2007; 50(22):2156–61.
25. Vanassche T, Lauw MN, Eikelboom JW, et al. Risk of ischaemic stroke according to pattern of atrial fibrillation: analysis of 6563 aspirin-treated patients in ACTIVE-A and AVERROES. Eur Heart J 2015;36(5):281–7a.
26. Vingerhoets F, Bogousslavsky J, Regli F, et al. Atrial fibrillation after acute stroke. Stroke 1993;24(1):26–30.
27. Gage BF, Waterman AD, Shannon W, et al. Validation of clinical classification schemes for predicting stroke: results from the National Registry of Atrial Fibrillation. JAMA 2001;285(22):2864–70.
28. Depta JP, Bhatt DL. Atherothrombosis and atrial fibrillation: important and often overlapping clinical syndromes. Thromb Haemost 2010;104(10):657–63.
29. European Heart Rhythm Association, European Association for Cardio-Thoracic Surgery, Camm AJ, Kirchhof P, Lip GYH, et al. Guidelines for the management of atrial fibrillation: the task force for the Management of Atrial Fibrillation of the European Society of Cardiology (ESC). Eur Heart J 2010;31(19):2369–429.
30. Lip GYH, Nieuwlaat R, Pisters R, et al. Refining clinical risk stratification for predicting stroke and thromboembolism in atrial fibrillation using a novel risk factor-based approach: the euro heart survey on atrial fibrillation. Chest 2010;137(2): 263–72.
31. Lip GYH, Frison L, Halperin JL, et al. Identifying patients at high risk for stroke despite anticoagulation: a comparison of contemporary stroke risk stratification schemes in an anticoagulated atrial fibrillation cohort. Stroke 2010;41(12): 2731–8.
32. van den Ham HA, Klungel OH, Singer DE, et al. Comparative performance of AT-RIA, CHADS2, and CHA2DS2-VASc risk scores predicting stroke in patients with atrial fibrillation: results from a National Primary Care Database. J Am Coll Cardiol 2015;66(17):1851–9.
33. Freedman B, Potpara TS, Lip GYH. Stroke prevention in atrial fibrillation. Lancet 2016;388(10046):806–17.
34. Hart RG, Pearce LA, Aguilar MI. Meta-analysis: antithrombotic therapy to prevent stroke in patients who have nonvalvular atrial fibrillation. Ann Intern Med 2007; 146(12):857–67.
35. Freedman B, Martinez C, Katholing A, et al. Residual risk of stroke and death in anticoagulant-treated patients with atrial fibrillation. JAMA Cardiol 2016;1(3): 366–8.
36. Active Investigators, Connolly SJ, Pogue J, Hart RG, et al. Effect of clopidogrel added to aspirin in patients with atrial fibrillation. N Engl J Med 2009;360(20): 2066 78.
37. ACTIVE Writing Group of the ACTIVE Investigators, Connolly S, Pogue J, Hart R, et al. Clopidogrel plus aspirin versus oral anticoagulation for atrial fibrillation in the Atrial fibrillation Clopidogrel Trial with Irbesartan for prevention of Vascular Events (ACTIVE W): a randomised controlled trial. Lancet 2006;367(9526):1903–12.
38. Lip GYH, Al-Khatib SM, Cosio FG, et al. Contemporary management of atrial fibrillation: what can clinical registries tell us about stroke prevention and current therapeutic approaches? J Am Heart Assoc 2014;3(4).

39. Kakkar AK, Mueller I, Bassand J-P, et al. Risk profiles and antithrombotic treatment of patients newly diagnosed with atrial fibrillation at risk of stroke: perspectives from the international, observational, prospective GARFIELD registry. PLoS One 2013;8(5):e63479.

40. Stangier J. Clinical pharmacokinetics and pharmacodynamics of the oral direct thrombin inhibitor dabigatran etexilate. Clin Pharmacokinet 2008;47(5):285–95.

41. Raghavan N, Frost CE, Yu Z, et al. Apixaban metabolism and pharmacokinetics after oral administration to humans. Drug Metab Dispos 2009;37(1):74–81.

42. Connolly SJ, Eikelboom J, Joyner C, et al. Apixaban in patients with atrial fibrillation. N Engl J Med 2011;364(9):806–17.

43. Siontis KC, Zhang X, Eckard A, et al. Outcomes associated with apixaban use in patients with end-stage kidney disease and atrial fibrillation in the United States. Circulation 2018;138(15):1519–29.

44. Giugliano RP, Ruff CT, Braunwald E, et al. Edoxaban versus warfarin in patients with atrial fibrillation. N Engl J Med 2013;369(22):2093–104.

45. Ruff CT, Giugliano RP, Braunwald E, et al. Association between edoxaban dose, concentration, anti-Factor Xa activity, and outcomes: an analysis of data from the randomised, double-blind ENGAGE AF-TIMI 48 trial. Lancet 2015;385(9984):2288–95.

46. Eriksson BI, Quinlan DJ, Weitz JI. Comparative pharmacodynamics and pharmacokinetics of oral direct thrombin and factor xa inhibitors in development. Clin Pharmacokinet 2009;48(1):1–22.

47. van Ryn J, Grottke O, Spronk H. Measurement of dabigatran in standardly used clinical assays, whole blood viscoelastic coagulation, and thrombin generation assays. Clin Lab Med 2014;34(3):479–501.

48. Dale BJ, Chan NC, Eikelboom JW. Laboratory measurement of the direct oral anticoagulants. Br J Haematol 2016;172(3):315–36.

49. Samuelson BT, Cuker A, Siegal DM, et al. Laboratory assessment of the anticoagulant activity of direct oral anticoagulants: a systematic review. Chest 2017;151(1):127–38.

50. Abstracts of the XXV congress of the International Society on Thrombosis and Haemostasis, June 20-25, 2015. J Thromb Haemost 2015;13(Suppl 2):1–997.

51. Schiele F, van Ryn J, Canada K, et al. A specific antidote for dabigatran: functional and structural characterization. Blood 2013;121(18):3554–62.

52. Pollack CV, Reilly PA, van Ryn J, et al. Idarucizumab for Dabigatran reversal - full cohort analysis. N Engl J Med 2017;377(5):431–41.

53. Connolly SJ, Milling TJ, Eikelboom JW, et al. Andexanet Alfa for acute major bleeding associated with factor Xa inhibitors. N Engl J Med 2016;375(12):1131–41.

54. Piran S, Khatib R, Schulman S, et al. Management of direct factor Xa inhibitor-related major bleeding with prothrombin complex concentrate: a meta-analysis. Blood adv 2019;3(2):158–67.

55. Fuster V, Rydén LE, Cannom DS, et al. 2011 ACCF/AHA/HRS focused updates incorporated into the ACC/AHA/ESC 2006 guidelines for the management of patients with atrial fibrillation: a report of the American College of Cardiology Foundation/American Heart Association Task Force on practice guidelines. Circulation 2011;123(10):e269–367.

56. De Caterina R, Camm AJ. What is "valvular" atrial fibrillation? A reappraisal. Eur Heart J 2014;35(47):3328–35.

57. Kannel WB, Wolf PA, Benjamin EJ, et al. Prevalence, incidence, prognosis, and predisposing conditions for atrial fibrillation: population-based estimates. Am J Cardiol 1998;82(8A):2N–9N.
58. Connolly SJ, Ezekowitz MD, Yusuf S, et al. Dabigatran versus warfarin in patients with atrial fibrillation. N Engl J Med 2009;361(12):1139–51.
59. Patel MR, Mahaffey KW, Garg J, et al. Rivaroxaban versus Warfarin in nonvalvular atrial fibrillation. N Engl J Med 2011;365(10):883–91.
60. Eikelboom JW, Connolly SJ, Brueckmann M, et al. Dabigatran versus warfarin in patients with mechanical heart valves. N Engl J Med 2013;369(13):1206–14.
61. Durães AR, de Souza Roriz P, de Almeida Nunes B, et al. Dabigatran versus warfarin after bioprosthesis valve replacement for the management of atrial fibrillation postoperatively: DAWA pilot study. Drugs R D 2016;16(2):149–54.
62. Pokorney Sean D, Rao Meena P, Wojdyla Daniel M, et al. Abstract 17277: apixaban use in patients with atrial fibrillation with bioprosthetic valves: insights from ARISTOTLE. Circulation 2015;132(suppl_3):A17277.
63. Mavrakanas TA, Samer CF, Nessim SJ, et al. Apixaban pharmacokinetics at steady state in hemodialysis patients. J Am Soc Nephrol 2017;28(7):2241–8.
64. Vázquez E, Sánchez-Perales C, Borrego F, et al. Influence of atrial fibrillation on the morbido-mortality of patients on hemodialysis. Am Heart J 2000;140(6): 886–90.
65. Marinigh R, Lane DA, Lip GYH. Severe renal impairment and stroke prevention in atrial fibrillation: implications for thromboprophylaxis and bleeding risk. J Am Coll Cardiol 2011;57(12):1339–48.
66. Reed D, Palkimas S, Hockman R, et al. Safety and effectiveness of apixaban compared to warfarin in dialysis patients. Res Pract Thromb Haemost 2018; 2(2):291–8.
67. Stanton BE, Barasch NS, Tellor KB. Comparison of the safety and effectiveness of apixaban versus warfarin in patients with severe renal impairment. Pharmacotherapy 2017;37(4):412–9.
68. Healey JS, Connolly SJ, Gold MR, et al. Subclinical atrial fibrillation and the risk of stroke. N Engl J Med 2012;366(2):120–9.
69. Glotzer TV, Daoud EG, Wyse DG, et al. The relationship between daily atrial tachyarrhythmia burden from implantable device diagnostics and stroke risk: the TRENDS study. Circ Arrhythm Electrophysiol 2009;2(5):474–80.
70. Verma A, Cairns JA, Mitchell LB, et al. 2014 focused update of the Canadian Cardiovascular Society Guidelines for the management of atrial fibrillation. Can J Cardiol 2014;30(10):1114–30.
71. January CT, Wann LS, Calkins H, et al. 2019 AHA/ACC/HRS focused update of the 2014 AHA/ACC/HRS guideline for the management of patients with atrial fibrillation: a report of the American College of Cardiology/American Heart Association Task Force on Clinical Practice Guidelines and the Heart Rhythm Society. Heart Rhythm 2019 [pii:S1547-5271(19)30037-2].
72. Lopes RD, Alings M, Connolly SJ, et al. Rationale and design of the Apixaban for the reduction of thrombo-embolism in patients with device-detected sub-clinical atrial fibrillation (ARTESiA) trial. Am Heart J 2017;189:137–45.
73. Manning WJ, Leeman DE, Gotch PJ, et al. Pulsed Doppler evaluation of atrial mechanical function after electrical cardioversion of atrial fibrillation. J Am Coll Cardiol 1989;13(3):617–23.
74. Gallagher MM, Hennessy BJ, Edvardsson N, et al. Embolic complications of direct current cardioversion of atrial arrhythmias: association with low intensity

of anticoagulation at the time of cardioversion. J Am Coll Cardiol 2002;40(5): 926–33.

75. Nagarakanti R, Ezekowitz MD, Oldgren J, et al. Dabigatran versus warfarin in patients with atrial fibrillation: an analysis of patients undergoing cardioversion. Circulation 2011;123(2):131–6.

76. Berger M, Schweitzer P. Timing of thromboembolic events after electrical cardioversion of atrial fibrillation or flutter: a retrospective analysis. Am J Cardiol 1998; 82(12):1545–7. A8.

77. Arnold AZ, Mick MJ, Mazurek RP, et al. Role of prophylactic anticoagulation for direct current cardioversion in patients with atrial fibrillation or atrial flutter. J Am Coll Cardiol 1992;19(4):851–5.

78. Granger CB, Alexander JH, McMurray JJV, et al. Apixaban versus warfarin in patients with atrial fibrillation. N Engl J Med 2011;365(11):981–92.

79. Botkin SB, Dhanekula LS, Olshansky B. Outpatient cardioversion of atrial arrhythmias: efficacy, safety, and costs. Am Heart J 2003;145(2):233–8.

80. Grönberg T, Hartikainen JEK, Nuotio I, et al. Anticoagulation, CHA2DS2VASc score, and thromboembolic risk of cardioversion of acute atrial fibrillation (from the FinCV Study). Am J Cardiol 2016;117(8):1294–8.

81. Melduni RM, Schaff HV, Lee H-C, et al. Impact of left atrial appendage closure during cardiac surgery on the occurrence of early postoperative atrial fibrillation, stroke, and mortality: a propensity score-matched analysis of 10 633 patients. Circulation 2017;135(4):366–78.

82. Cappato R, Ezekowitz MD, Klein AL, et al. Rivaroxaban vs. vitamin K antagonists for cardioversion in atrial fibrillation. Eur Heart J 2014;35(47):3346–55.

83. Ezekowitz MD, Pollack CV, Halperin JL, et al. Apixaban compared to heparin/ vitamin K antagonist in patients with atrial fibrillation scheduled for cardioversion: the EMANATE trial. Eur Heart J 2018;39(32):2959–71.

Supraventricular Tachycardia

Arun Umesh Mahtani, MBBS[1], Devi Gopinath Nair, MD, FHRS*

KEYWORDS

- Tachycardia • Supraventricular arrhythmias • Cardiac heart diseases
- Accessory pathways • AVNRT • Radio frequency ablation

KEY POINTS

- The term paroxysmal supraventricular tachycardia encompasses a heterogeneous group of arrhythmias with different electrophysiologic characteristics.
- Knowledge of the mechanism of each supraventricular tachycardia is important in determining management in the office, at the bedside, and in the electrophysiology laboratory.
- Such paroxysmal supraventricular tachycardias have an abrupt onset and offset, typically initiating and terminating with premature atrial ectopic beats.
- In the acute setting, both vagal maneuvers and pharmacologic therapy can be effective in arrhythmia termination.
- Catheter ablation has revolutionized therapy for many supraventricular tachycardias, and newer techniques have significantly improved ablation efficacy and reduced periprocedural complications and procedure times.

Supraventricular tachycardia (SVT) is a common term used to describe tachycardias with rates of more than 100 bpm, with a mechanism that involves the atrial tissue up to the atrioventricular junction (AVJ). These include atrioventricular nodal reentrant tachycardia (AVNRT), various types of accessory pathway-mediated atrioventricular reentrant tachycardias (AVRT), atrial tachycardia (AT), including focal and multifocal mechanisms, sinus tachycardia, atrial flutter, and atrial fibrillation. Paroxysmal SVT (PSVT) is the term used for a subset of SVTs that have an abrupt onset and offset such as AVNRT, AVRT, and AT. The prevalence of SVT in the general population is 2.29 per 1000 persons.[1] When adjusted by age and sex in the US population, the incidence of PSVT is estimated to be 36 per 100,000 persons per year. Compared with

Disclosure Statement: The authors have no financial relationships to disclose pertaining to the content of this article.

Department of Cardiac Electrophysiology, St. Bernard's Heart and Vascular Center, Jonesboro, AR, USA

[1] Present address: Unit B-306, Mantri Elegance Apartments, Bannerghatta Road, Bangalore, Karnataka 560076, India.

* Corresponding author. 3878 Ridgewood Cv, Jonesboro, AR 72404.

E-mail address: drdevignair@gmail.com

Med Clin N Am 103 (2019) 863–879
https://doi.org/10.1016/j.mcna.2019.05.007
0025-7125/19/© 2019 Elsevier Inc. All rights reserved.

medical.theclinics.com

patients with cardiovascular disease, those with PSVT without cardiovascular disease are younger (37 vs 69 years; $P = .0002$) and have faster PSVT (186 bpm vs 155 bpm; $P = .0006$). Women have twice the risk of men of developing PSVT.[1] Individuals greater than 65 years of age have more than 5 times the risk of younger persons of developing PSVT.[1]

AVNRT is more common in persons who are middle aged or older, whereas in adolescents, the prevalence may be more balanced between AVRT and AVNRT, or AVRT may be more prevalent.[1] The relative frequency of tachycardia mediated by an accessory pathway decreases with age. The incidence of manifest preexcitation or a Wolff–Parkinson–White syndrome pattern on electrocardiogram (ECG) tracings in the general population is 0.1% to 0.3%. However, not all patients with manifest ventricular preexcitation develop PSVT.[2–4]

CLASSIFICATION

There are different ways of classifying PSVT.

Based on site of origin
a. Impulse originating from the atrial tissue above the AVJ, without using the AVJ as part of the circuit:
   Rhythms in this category include atrial fibrillation, AT, atrial flutter with variable conduction, or multifocal AT (MAT).
b. Impulse using AVJ as part of circuit:
   Rhythms in this category include AVNRT, AVRT, and junctional tachycardia.

Based on the RP interval (the RP interval is the interval between the onset of a surface QRS to the onset of a visible P wave).
a. No RP tachycardia with no visible P waves:
   Rhythms in this category include Typical AVNRT and AT.
b. Very short RP interval tachycardia with the RP interval of less than or equal to the PR interval and the actual RP interval less than 90 ms:
   Rhythms in this category include typical AVNRT and AT.
c. Short RP interval tachycardia with the RP interval of less than or equal to the PR interval and the actual RP interval is 90 ms or greater:
   Rhythms in this category include orthodromic AVRT, atypical AVNRT, and AT.
d. Long RP interval tachycardia where the RP interval is greater than or equal to the PR interval: rhythms in this category include sinus tachycardia, AT, permanent junctional reciprocating tachycardia, and atypical AVNRT.

An algorithm for the differential diagnosis of PSVT is shown in **Fig. 1**.

MECHANISMS OF DIFFERENT TYPES OF PAROXYSMAL SUPRAVENTRICULAR TACHYCARDIA
Atrioventricular Nodal Reentrant Tachycardia

AVNRT accounts for most of the cases of PSVT.[5] It is most commonly seen in women who are in their fourth or fifth decade of life.[6,7]

AVNRT occurs in patients who exhibit dual atrioventricular nodal physiology with a slow pathway and a fast pathway within the atrioventricular node (AVN). The slow pathway has a slow conduction velocity but a relatively shorter refractory period, whereas the fast pathway has a swift conduction velocity, but a significantly longer refractory period. Conduction through these 2 pathways can either be in the anterograde or retrograde direction.[8–10]

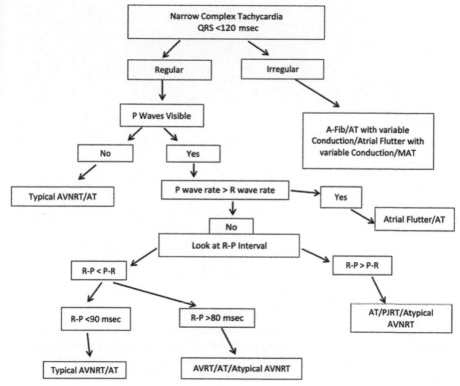

Fig. 1. Algorithm for differential diagnosis of narrow complex tachycardia. A-Fib, atrial fibrillation; PJRT, permanent junctional reciprocating tachycardia.

Typical Atrioventricular Nodal Reentrant Tachycardia

In sinus rhythm, the impulse is conducted from the atrium to the ventricles through the fast pathway of the AVN and through the bundle of His. Typical AVNRT begins when there is a perfectly timed premature atrial depolarization that blocks in the fast pathway during its refractory state and propagates through the slow pathway in the AVN, reaching the ventricles. However, if the propagation is slow enough and the fast pathway comes out of its refractory state, the impulse can travel retrograde into the atria creating a reentry circuit within the AVN. The antegrade limb of the circuit is down the slow pathway and the retrograde limb of the circuit is up the fast pathway. The atria and ventricles are depolarized simultaneously as bystanders and do not participate in the tachycardia.

Electrocardiogram characteristics of typical atrioventricular nodal reentrant tachycardia

As the first premature impulse travels over the slow pathway in the antegrade direction, there is evidence of a prolonged PR interval in the initiating beat of the tachycardia. During reentry, there is simultaneous activation of the atria and ventricles. Hence, the P wave and the QRS complex occur almost simultaneously resulting in a no RP or very short RP tachycardia (**Fig. 2**). The P wave will be negative in leads II, II, and aVF as the impulse travels retrograde from the low to the high atrium. The P waves also have smaller width suggesting septal activation.

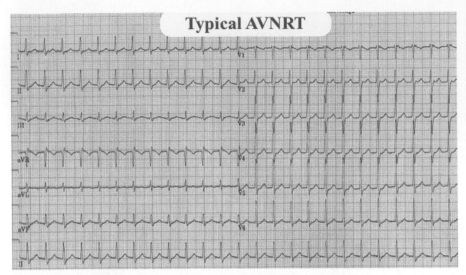

Fig. 2. ECG of a typical AVNRT, with a very short RP/no RP tachycardia.

Atypical Atrioventricular Nodal Reentrant Tachycardia

There is a role reversal in atypical AVNRT. A perfectly timed premature ventricular depolarization activates the slow pathway in a retrograde fashion, depolarizing the atria; the ventricles are activated thereafter through the fast pathway in an antegrade fashion. Atypical AVNRT occurs in about 10% of all patients having AVNRT.[6]

Electrocardiogram characteristics of atypical atrioventricular nodal reentrant tachycardia

In atypical AVNRT there is a clear separation between the P waves and the QRS complexes. Tachycardia is usually initiated by a premature atrial or ventricular contraction. The PR interval is normal as the impulse travels antegrade through the fast pathway, as it would in sinus rhythm. However, the RP interval, which represents retrograde conduction of the electrical signal through the slow pathway, is prolonged, resulting in a long RP tachycardia. The P wave continues to remain negative in leads II, III, and aVF as the impulse travels in the atrium from bottom to top, and the vector is therefore directed away from these leads (**Figs. 3** and **4**). The P waves also have smaller width, suggesting septal activation.

Atrioventricular Reentrant Tachycardia

AVRT is the second most common PSVT in clinical practice,[5] usually seen in a younger population.[9] In AVRT, the circuit includes the AVN and an accessory pathway connecting the atria and ventricles that allows for antegrade and/or retrograde conduction.

An accessory pathway is an abnormal band of conducting tissue that can transmit impulses anterograde, retrograde, and or both. When an impulse is transmitted anterograde across this pathway,[9] the region of the ventricle connected to this pathway is excited/depolarized earlier than the rest of the ventricle, known as ventricular preexcitation, resulting in the characteristic delta wave and a short PR interval. This type of pathway is called a "manifest" pathway, because it is clearly visible while in sinus rhythm. Manifest accessory pathways can conduct retrograde as well. Accessory

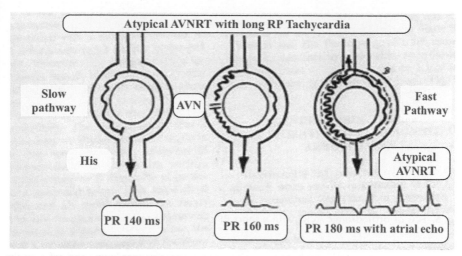

Fig. 3. Initiation of atypical AVNRT.

pathways that can only conduct impulses in a retrograde direction are called "concealed" accessory pathways, because there is no ventricular preexcitation and no evidence of ECG changes while in sinus rhythm.[11,12]

Orthodromic Atrioventricular Nodal Reentrant Tachycardia

This is the most common mechanism of AVRT among patients with accessory pathway.[13] It starts with a perfectly timed premature atrial contraction that travels through the AVN and the His-Purkinje system to cause ventricular depolarization. The impulse then travels retrograde through the accessory pathway to the atria forming a reentrant circuit.

Electrocardiogram characteristics of orthodromic atrioventricular nodal reentrant tachycardia

Tachycardia is usually initiated by a premature atrial or ventricular contraction. During reentry, there is activation of the ventricles through the AVN in an antegrade fashion,

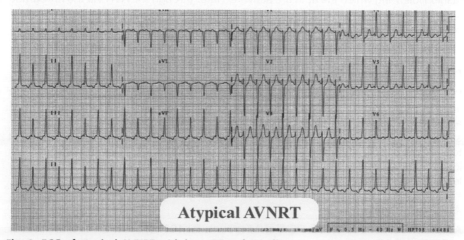

Fig. 4. ECG of atypical AVNRT with long RP tachycardia.

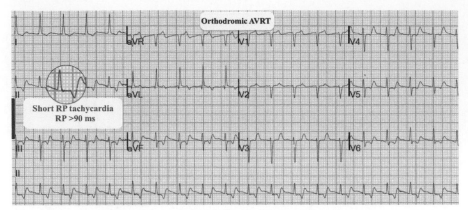

Fig. 5. ECG of orthodromic AVRT with a short RP (RP >80 ms) tachycardia.

resulting in a narrow QRS tachycardia, after which the atria are activated retrograde through the accessory pathway. Hence, the P wave follows the QRS complex resulting in a short RP (much less frequently a long RP) depending on the site and conduction properties of the accessory pathway. The P wave morphology depends on the site of the accessory pathway (**Fig. 5**).

Antidromic Atrioventricular Nodal Reentrant Tachycardia

This entity is rare compared with orthodromic AVRT and is usually seen in about 10% of the patients with manifest accessory pathway.[14–21] Here, the premature impulse travels anterograde through the accessory pathway and reentry into the atria is via the Hisian system and the AVN. It is more common among patients with multiple accessory pathways.[15]

Electrocardiogram characteristics of antidromic atrioventricular nodal reentrant tachycardia

Tachycardia is usually initiated by a premature atrial or ventricular contraction. During reentry, there is activation of the ventricles by the accessory pathway in the antegrade fashion following which the atria are activated later through the AVN via the retrograde approach. Owing to the maximum preexcitation of the ventricles, this is a wide complex tachycardia and the QRS morphology depends on the site of the accessory pathway (**Fig. 6**).

Permanent Junctional Reciprocating Tachycardia

Permanent junctional reciprocating tachycardia is a type of orthodromic AVRT usually seen in pediatric population or young adults using a slowly conducting concealed accessory pathway. Permanent junctional reciprocating tachycardia is usually incessant[22] and if left untreated, patients will have a deterioration of cardiac function owing to cardiomyopathy that can ultimately lead to heart failure.[23] This pattern results in a long RP tachycardia with a P wave morphology that is typically negative in the inferior leads, but varies depending on the location of the accessory pathway.

Atrial Tachycardia

AT is the least common of the PSVTs. It accounts for 10% of the total number of cases of PSVT.[24,25] AT originates in the atrial tissue and does not require another part of the

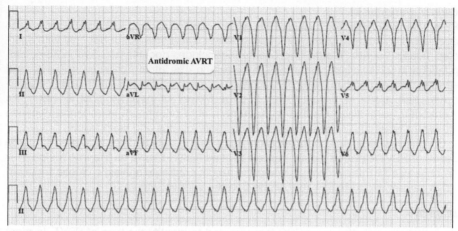

Fig. 6. ECG of antidromic AVRT; wide complex tachycardia with maximum preexcitation.

conduction system for its propagation. There are 2 types of AT that can cause SVT, unifocal AT and MAT.

Unifocal Atrial Tachycardia

In unifocal AT, the electrical impulse originates from one site located anywhere in the atria. The P wave pattern on the ECG depends on the site of origin of the ectopic impulse. The patient could have 1:1 AV conduction or there could be more atrial impulses than ventricular impulses. Unifocal AT can be due to reentry or enhanced automaticity within an atrial focus. AT occurring owing to reentry is usually paroxysmal and is associated with underlying structural heart disease.[26] In contrast, enhanced automaticity is incessant and can occur in the setting of a structurally normal heart.[26] Treating the incessant variety is of utmost importance as failure to treat can lead to tachyarrhythmia-associated cardiomyopathy and ultimately heart failure.

Multifocal Atrial Tachycardia

In MAT, there are multiple foci located in the atria that have enhanced automaticity.[27] The diagnosis of MAT is usually based on an ECG criterion. It requires 3 or more different P wave morphologies, each representing a separate atrial focus, along with an average heart rate 100 beats per minute or more. Unlike atrial fibrillation, MAT has the presence of isoelectric periods between P waves. A wandering atrial pacemaker has a similar ECG appearance. The only difference is that the average heart rate is 100 beats per minute or less. A strong association has been found between MAT and various pulmonary diseases.[27]

Rare Types of Permanent Junctional Reciprocating Tachycardia

Sinoatrial reentrant tachycardia

Sinoatrial reentrant tachycardia is a rare cause of PSVT with a reentrant circuit originating within the sinus node.[28–31] Because the reentrant circuit is in the sinus node the P wave morphology remains identical to a normal sinus P wave. The only way to identify SART is to look for a prolonged RP interval when compared with a PR interval. In contrast with inappropriate sinus tachycardia, which is an automatic tachycardia, sinoatrial reentrant tachycardia starts and stops abruptly.

Clinical presentation

PSVTs have an impact on quality of life, which varies according to the frequency of the episodes, the duration of the SVT, and whether symptoms occur not only with exercise ,but also at rest. Modes of presentation includes documented SVT in 38%, palpitations in 22%, chest pain in 5%, syncope in 4%, atrial fibrillation in 0.4%, and sudden cardiac death in 0.2%.[32] PSVT is often misdiagnosed as panic or anxiety disorder, particularly in patients with a prior history of psychological illness.[33] As mentioned, early diagnosis and management is of paramount importance because incessant types of SVT can progress to cardiomyopathy and heart failure.

On physical examination tachycardia may be the only finding. However, in some cases of PSVT elevated jugular venous pressure also known as the frog's sign may be observed.[32] This sign occurs when the atrium contracts against a closed tricuspid valve causing blood to flow retrograde into the venous system.

Diagnosis

As with every arrhythmia, an ECG is warranted to identify the type of PSVT. In most cases of PSVT the QRS complex is narrow. However, wide QRS complexes can occasionally be seen.[34] It is important to look for characteristics like P wave morphology, QRS morphology, PR interval, and RP interval. Clinically, this is important because the treatment options vary for each type of PSVT. Other investigations to consider are an echocardiogram to look for underlying structural heart disease, electrolyte abnormalities, and serum thyroid-stimulating hormone levels because they can all be triggers for the PSVT. The importance of pulmonary disease in the setting of a structurally normal heart should be emphasized. Patients with many pulmonary diseases, including asthma, chronic obstructive disease, and obstructive disease, are at a higher risk of developing atrial tachyarrhythmias. Cardiac monitoring, including continuous ambulatory monitoring using an external or implantable monitor, is sometimes required to capture the PSVT. Occasionally an invasive electrophysiological study might be required, usually in conjunction with a planned ablation treatment strategy.

Treatment Options

There are a wide variety of acute and long-term treatment options available to stop and eventually treat the PSVT.

ACUTE MANAGEMENT OPTIONS
Nonpharmacologic Methods

Nonpharmacologic treatment is usually the first step to control a PSVT episode when there is no hemodynamic instability. The principle behind nonpharmacologic methods is to increase vagal tone, which in turn slows conduction through the AVN. Because a majority of PSVTs use the AVN as part of their reentry circuit, such maneuvers can terminate the reentrant circuit. This method of treatment can also be used to diagnose the type of PSVT[35,36]:

a. *The Valsalva maneuver* is an effective way to abort an episode of PSVT. This method was first described in the year 1936 by Hamilton and continues to remain an effective method to stop an episode of PSVT. This can be done by bearing down, coughing, or splashing cold water over the face.
b. *Carotid sinus massage*: The carotid sinus is an area in the carotid artery that has pressure-sensitive receptors to maintain adequate blood pressure and control cardiac output. It is found just below the angle of the jaw. Massaging over this area for 10 seconds causes firing of these pressure-sensitive receptors and causes a

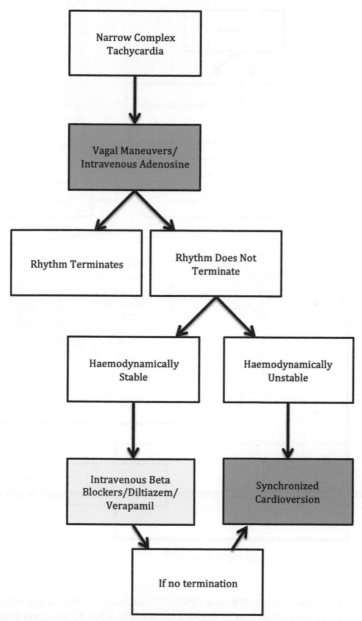

Fig. 7. Algorithm for the acute treatment of narrow complex tachycardia.

vagally induced slowing of conduction through the AVN. Precautions while performing this maneuver include performing it only over 1 side and avoiding it in elderly patients with audible carotid bruits.[35]

Pharmacologic Methods

Pharmacologic therapy for acute termination of PSVT is appropriate when nonpharmacologic maneuvers fail. The preferred initial agents are intravenous adenosine or

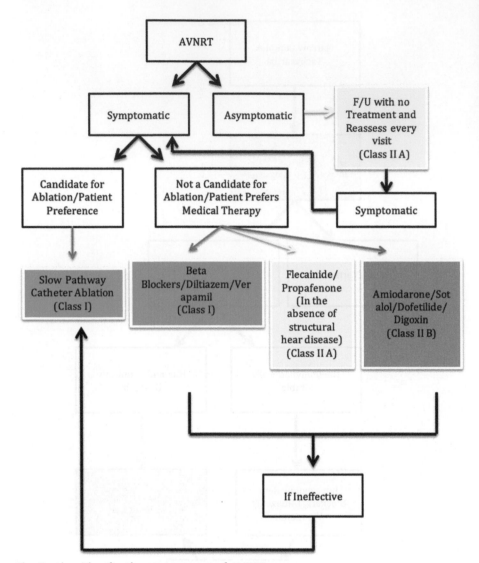

Fig. 8. Algorithm for the management of AVNRT.

a nondihydropyridine calcium channel blocker. Adenosine's effects are mediated by membrane hyperpolarization that typically occurs within 15 to 30 seconds after administration. Adenosine has a powerful effect on the AVN and is highly effective in causing transient, complete AVN block. Transient sinus bradycardia or sinus arrests often occur but are short lived. The ECG should be recorded continuously during adenosine administration to document the effect of the drug on PSVT and to monitor for the rare occurrence of proarrhythmia. Patients should be warned that they might experience short-lived sensations of claustrophobia, dyspnea, flushing, and chest discomfort. The initial dose of adenosine is 6 mg intravenous bolus (flushed), using a large vein. Subsequent doses of 12 mg or even 18-mg boluses may be required. PSVT resolution after adenosine administration establishes AVNRT or AVRT as the likely PSVT

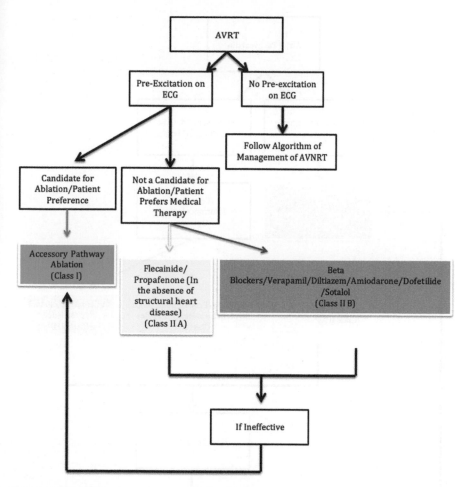

Fig. 9. Algorithm for the management of AVRT.

mechanism, although occasionally unifocal AT will terminate with adenosine as well. In most unifocal ATs, adenosine administration results in a transient slowing of the ventricular rate, revealing the underlying atrial activity. Adenosine should be used carefully in patients with Wolff–Parkinson–White syndrome and atrial fibrillation because it shortens the refractory period of the accessory pathway resulting in rapid conduction of atrial fibrillation, increasing the chances of dangerous ventricular tachyarrhythmias from preexcited atrial fibrillation. Etripamil in the form of a nasal spray is a short acting calcium channel blocker and has been tested for acute termination of PSVT episodes. The rates of conversion to sinus rhythm are high and the time to conversion is less than 3 minutes, with a low side effect profile.

The use of direct current cardioversion is generally limited to cases of hemodynamically unstable PSVT that do not respond to any of these methods and is a rare phenomenon.[37] An algorithm for the acute management of PSVT is presented in **Fig. 7**.

Long-Term Management

Referral to an electrophysiologist is indicated for patients with poorly tolerated or frequently recurring arrhythmias. Most of the time, patients with AVNRT or AVRT are

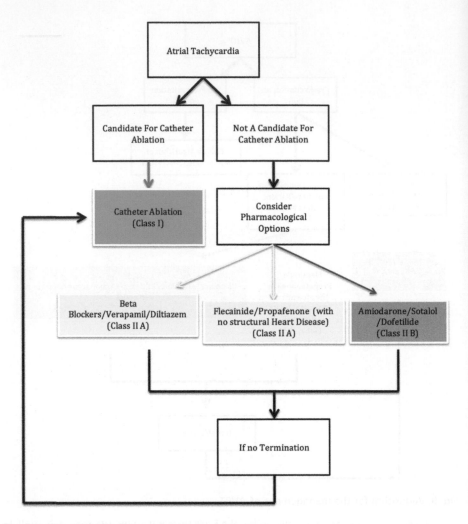

Fig. 10. Algorithm for the management of AT.

referred for ablation before extended trials of drug therapy because these rhythms are curable at least 95% of the time.

Pharmacologic Treatment

Chronic prophylactic drug therapy is an important treatment option for patients with PSVT who have difficulty self-terminating their arrhythmia. Patient age, frequency of PSVT, and symptom burden should all be taken into account before considering chronic prophylactic medical therapy. Pharmacotherapy is associated with side effects and often does not result in complete freedom from arrhythmia.

Both long-acting calcium channel blockers and beta blockers improve symptoms in 60 to 80% of patients with PSVT.[38,39] Flecainide and propafenone are class IC antiarrhythmic drugs that suppress automaticity and slow conduction and can thus result in a significant decrease in duration and frequency of PSVT episodes. These drugs are

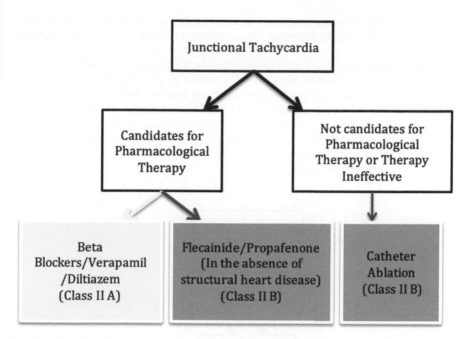

Fig. 11. Algorithm for the management of junctional tachycardia.

contraindicated in patients with known structural heart disease because of an increased risk of ventricular arrhythmias.[39,40]

Class III drugs such as sotalol or dofetilide are also effective in controlling PSVT. These drugs prolong the refractory period, prevent propagation of reentry, and suppress automaticity.[41] Class III antiarrhythmic drugs carry the risk of long QT and Torsades de Pointes and must be managed by an electrophysiologist. In fact, most electrophysiologists would recommend a catheter ablation before antiarrhythmic drug therapy for the vast majority of PSVTs, save for atrial fibrillation. This recommendation is because antiarrhythmic drugs expose the patient to the real risk of proarrhythmia over the long term, in addition to other noncardiac side effects.

Catheter Ablation

Given the high success rates and favorable safety profiles of diagnostic electrophysiology study followed by catheter ablation, many patients choose this option early in their course. Guidelines recommend ablation for patients with recurrent PSVT based on the type of SVT and known success rates.[42] Complications of ablation for PSVT are generally low, although they vary significantly depending on the arrhythmia being treated. One large multicenter study examining patients undergoing AVNRT, AVRT, and AVN ablation found low risks of death, stroke, myocardial infarction, tamponade, and arterial perforation. Procedures involving ablation near the AVN are more likely to be complicated by atrioventricular block. Other possible complications include pericardial and pleural effusions, pneumothorax, and damage to the coronary vasculature and valves, although these complications are rare.[42]

Ablation of AVNRT targets the slow pathway of the AVN, located along the posterior tricuspid annulus near the coronary sinus ostium. Slow pathway modification using radiofrequency ablation or cryoablation results in success rate of 99% for the permanent cure of AVNRT (**Fig. 8**). However, the incidence of complete heart block remains 1.0% to 1.5%.[43,44]

Success rates for accessory pathway ablation for the treatment of AVRT range from 95% to 98%, with recurrence rates of AVRT as low as 2% (**Fig. 9**). Location of the accessory pathway can have a significant effect on success rates,[45,46] with accurate localization of the accessory pathway being key to a successful procedure.

Unifocal AT ablation is indicated in patients with recurrent, symptomatic episodes. The use of 3-dimensional mapping technology has significantly improved the efficacy of focal AT ablation with success rates ranging from 69% to 100%,[47] with recurrence rates as low as 8% (**Figs. 10–12**).

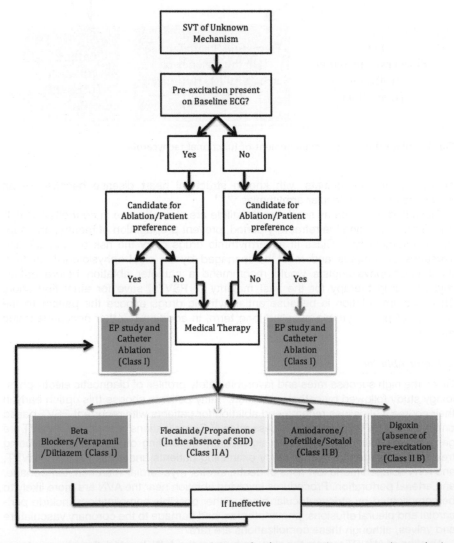

Fig. 12. Algorithm for the management of PSVT of unknown mechanism. EP, electrophysiologic; SHD, structural heart disease.

SUMMARY

PSVT encompasses a heterogeneous group of arrhythmias with different electrophysiologic characteristics. Knowledge of the mechanism of each SVT is important in determining management in the office, at the bedside, and in the electrophysiology laboratory. In the acute setting, both vagal maneuvers and pharmacologic therapy can be effective in arrhythmia termination. Catheter ablation has revolutionized therapy for many SVTs, and newer techniques have significantly improved ablation efficacy and reduced periprocedural complications and procedure times.

REFERENCES

1. Orejarena LA, Vidaillet H Jr, DeStefano F, et al. Paroxysmal supraventricular tachycardia in the general population. J Am Coll Cardiol 1998;31(1):150–7.
2. Lu C-W, Wu M-H, Chen H-C, et al. Epidemiological profile of Wolff-Parkinson-White syndrome in a general population younger than 50 years of age in an era of radiofrequency catheter ablation. Int J Cardiol 2014;174:530–4.
3. Whinnett ZI, Sohaib SMA, Davies DW. Diagnosis and management of supraventricular tachycardia. BMJ 2012;345:e7769.
4. Porter MJ, Morton JB, Denman R, et al. Influence of age and gender on the mechanism of supraventricular tachycardia. Heart Rhythm 2004;1:393–6.
5. Wellens HJJ. 25 years of insights into the mechanisms of supraventricular arrhythmias: NASPE HISTORY SERIES. Pacing Clin Electrophysiol 2003;26(9): 1916–22.
6. Akhtar M, Jazayeri MR, Sra J, et al. Atrioventricular nodal reentry. Clinical, electrophysiological, and therapeutic considerations. Circulation 1993;88(1):282–95.
7. Jazayeri MR, Hempe SL, Sra JS, et al. Selective transcatheter ablation of the fast and slow pathways using radiofrequency energy in patients with atrioventricular nodal reentrant tachycardia. Circulation 1992;85(4):1318–28.
8. Ganz LI, Friedman PL. Supraventricular tachycardia. N Engl J Med 1995;332(3): 162–73.
9. Link MS. Evaluation and initial treatment of supraventricular tachycardia. N Engl J Med 2012;367(15):1438–48.
10. Brugada P, Bär FW, Vanagt EJ, et al. Observations in patients showing AV junctional echoes with a shorter PR than RP interval: distinction between intranodal reentry or reentry using an accessory pathway with a long conduction time. Am J Cardiol 1981;48(4):611–22.
11. Oren JW, Beckman KJ, McClelland JH, et al. A functional approach to the preexcitation syndromes. Cardiol Clin 1993;11(1):121–49.
12. Wolff L. Bundle branch block with short PR interval in healthy young people prone to paroxysmal tachycardia. Am Heart J 1930;5:685–704.
13. Josephson ME. Clinical cardiac electrophysiology: techniques and interpretations. Lippincott Williams & Wilkins; 2008. Available at: https://scholar.google. com/scholar?hl=en&as_sdt=0%2C36&q=Josephson+ME.+Clinical+cardiac+ electrophysiology%3A+techniques+and+interpretations.+Lippincott+Williams+ %26+Wilkins%3B+2008.&btnG=.
14. Bardy GH, Packer DL, German LD, et al. Preexcited reciprocating tachycardia in patients with Wolff-Parkinson-White syndrome: incidence and mechanisms. Circulation 1984;70(3):377–91.
15. Ati J, Brugada P, Brugada J, et al. Clinical and electrophysiologic characteristics of patients with antidromic circus movement tachycardia in the Wolff-Parkinson-White syndrome. Am J Cardiol 1990;66(15):1082–91.

16. Campbell RWF, Smith RA, Gallagher JJ, et al. Atrial fibrillation in the preexcitation syndrome. Am J Cardiol 1977;40(4):514–20. https://www.ncbi.nlm.nih.gov/pubmed/?term=Pritchett%20EL%5BAuthor%5D&cauthor=true&cauthor_uid=910715.
17. Klein GJ, Bashore TM, Sellers TD, et al. Ventricular fibrillation in the Wolff-Parkinson-White syndrome. N Engl J Med 1979;301(20):1080–5.
18. Torner P, Brugada P, Smeets J, et al. Ventricular fibrillation in the Wolff-Parkinson-White syndrome. Eur Heart J 1991;12(2):144–50.
19. Morady F, Sledge C, Shen E, et al. Electrophysiologic testing in the management of patients with the Wolff-Parkinson-White syndrome and atrial fibrillation. Am J Cardiol 1983;51(10):1623–8.
20. Wellens HJ, Braat S, Brugada P, et al. Use of procainamide in patients with the Wolff-Parkinson-White syndrome to disclose a short refractory period of the accessory pathway. Am J Cardiol 1982;50(5):1087–9.
21. Strasberg B, Ashley WW, Wyndham CR, et al. Treadmill exercise testing in the Wolff-Parkinson-White syndrome. Am J Cardiol 1980;45(4):742–8.
22. Farré J, Ross D, Wiener I, et al. Reciprocal tachycardias using accessory pathways with long conduction times. Dordrecht (the Netherlands): Springer; 2000. p. 197–213. Professor Hein JJ Wellens.
23. Cruz FES, Cheriex EC, Smeets JL, et al. Reversibility of tachycardia-induced cardiomyopathy after cure of incessant supraventricular tachycardia. J Am Coll Cardiol 1990;16(3):739–44.
24. Chen S-A, Chiang CE, Yang CJ, et al. Sustained atrial tachycardia in adult patients. Electrophysiological characteristics, pharmacological response, possible mechanisms, and effects of radiofrequency ablation. Circulation 1994;90(3):1262–78.
25. Kistler PM, Roberts-Thomson KC, Haqqani HM, et al. P-wave morphology in focal atrial tachycardia: development of an algorithm to predict the anatomic site of origin. J Am Coll Cardiol 2006;48(5):1010–7.
26. Haines DE, DiMarco JP. Sustained intraatrial reentrant tachycardia: clinical, electrocardiographic and electrophysiologic characteristics and long-term follow-up. J Am Coll Cardiol 1990;15(6):1345–54.
27. Kastor JA. Multifocal atrial tachycardia. N Engl J Med 1990;322(24):1713–7.
28. Wu D, Amat-y-leon F, Denes P, et al. Demonstration of sustained sinus and atrial re-entry as a mechanism of paroxysmal supraventricular tachycardia. Circulation 1975;51(2):234–43.
29. Rosen MR, Fisch C, Hoffman BF, et al. Can accelerated atrioventricular junctional escape rhythms be explained by delayed afterdepolarizations? Am J Cardiol 1980;45(6):1272–84.
30. Rosen KM. Junctional tachycardia: mechanisms, diagnosis, differential diagnosis, and management. Circulation 1973;47(3):654–64.
31. Colucci RA, Silver MJ, Shubrook J. Common types of supraventricular tachycardia: diagnosis and management. Am Fam Physician 2010;82(8):942–52.
32. Lessmeier TJ, Gamperling D, Johnson-Liddon V, et al. Unrecognized paroxysmal supraventricular tachycardia: potential for misdiagnosis as panic disorder. Arch Intern Med 1997;157(5):537–43.
33. Zimetbaum P, Josephson ME. Evaluation of patients with palpitations. N Engl J Med 1998;338(19):1369–73.
34. Antunes E, Brugada J, Steurer G, et al. The differential diagnosis of a regular tachycardia with a wide QRS complex on the 12-lead ECG: ventricular tachycardia, supraventricular tachycardia with aberrant intraventricular conduction,

and supraventricular tachycardia with anterograde conduction over an accessory pathway. Pacing Clin Electrophysiol 1994;17(9):1515–24.

35. Adlington H, Cumberbatch G. Carotid sinus massage: is it a safe way to terminate supraventricular tachycardia? Emerg Med J 2009;26(6):459.

36. Nishimura RA, Tajik AJ. The Valsalva maneuver and response revisited. Mayo Clin Proc 1986;61(3):211–7. Elsevier.

37. Stambler BS, Dorian P, Sager PT, et al. Etripamil nasal spray for rapid conversion of supraventricular tachycardia to sinus rhythm. J Am Coll Cardiol 2018;72(5): 489–97.

38. Lévy S, Ricard P. Using the right drug: a treatment algorithm for regular supraventricular tachycardias. Eur Heart J 1997;18(Suppl C):C27–32.

39. Dorian P, Naccarelli GV, Coumel P, et al. A randomized comparison of flecainide versus verapamil in paroxysmal supraventricular tachycardia. The Flecainide Multicenter Investigators Group. Am J Cardiol 1996;77(3):89A–95A.

40. UK Propafenone PSVT Study Group. A randomized, placebo-controlled trial of propafenone in the prophylaxis of paroxysmal supraventricular tachycardia and paroxysmal atrial fibrillation. Circulation 1995;92(9):2550–7.

41. Touboul P, Atallah G, Kirkorian G, et al. Effects of intravenous sotalol in patients with atrioventricular accessory pathways. Am Heart J 1987;114(3):545–50.

42. Calkins H, Yong P, Miller JM, et al. Catheter ablation of accessory pathways, atrioventricular nodal reentrant tachycardia, and the atrioventricular junction: final results of a prospective, multicenter clinical trial. The Atakr Multicenter Investigators Group. Circulation 1999;99(2):262–70.

43. Epstein LM, Lesh MD, Griffin JC, et al. A direct midseptal approach to slow atrioventricular nodal pathway ablation. Pacing Clin Electrophysiol 1995;18(1 Pt 1): 57–64.

44. Tanaka S, Yoshida A, Fukuzawa K, et al. Recognition of inferiorly dislocated fast pathways guided by three-dimensional electro-anatomical mapping. J Interv Card Electrophysiol 2011;32(2):95–103.

45. Friedman PL, Dubuc M, Green MS, et al. Catheter cryoablation of supraventricular tachycardia: results of the multicenter prospective "frosty" trial. Heart Rhythm 2004;1(2):129–38.

46. Hamilton K, Castillo M, Arruda M, et al. Echocardiographic demonstration of coronary sinus diverticula in patients with Wolff-Parkinson-White syndrome. J Am Soc Echocardiogr 1996;9(3):337–43.

47. Roberts-Thomson KC, Kistler PM, Kalman JM. Focal atrial tachycardia II: management. Pacing Clin Electrophysiol 2006;29(7):769–78.

Ventricular Arrhythmias

Soufian T. AlMahameed, MD*, Ohad Ziv, MD

KEYWORDS

- Ventricular tachycardia • Premature ventricular complexes
- Classification of ventricular arrhythmias

KEY POINTS

- Ventricular tachycardia is commonly seen in medical practice. It may be completely benign or portend a high risk for sudden cardiac death.
- It is of paramount importance that clinicians are familiar with and able to promptly recognize and manage ventricular tachycardia when confronted with it clinically.
- In many cases, curative therapy for a given ventricular arrhythmia may be provided after a thorough understanding of the underlying substrate and mechanism.

INTRODUCTION

Ventricular tachycardia (VT) is commonly seen in medical practice. It may be completely benign or portend high risk for sudden cardiac death (SCD). Therefore, it is of paramount importance that clinicians be familiar with and able to promptly recognize and manage VT when confronted with it clinically. In this article, we broadly review the current classification of the different ventricular arrhythmias encountered in medical practice, provide brief background regarding the different mechanisms, and discuss practical diagnosis and management scenarios.

Premature ventricular complexes (PVCs) refer to any cardiac rhythm that originates from below the atrioventricular node, whether it is a single complex or multiple consecutive complexes (**Fig. 1**A). These can originate from ventricular myocytes or from His-Purkinje tissue. A series of more than 3 consecutive PVCs at a rate faster than 100 beat per minute is referred to as VT. A series of more than 3 consecutive PVCs at a rate of less than 100 beat per minutes is referred to as an accelerated idioventricular rhythm. Monomorphic VT (MMVT) describes VT with a uniform QRS appearance, where every beat appears the same as the next on telemetry or electrocardiography (ECG) tracings (**Fig. 1**D, E). Polymorphic VT (PMVT), in contrast,

Disclosure Statement: The authors have nothing to disclose.
Heart and Vascular Research Center, MetroHealth Campus of Case Western Reserve University, 2500 MetroHealth Medical Drive, Cleveland, OH 44109, USA
* Corresponding author.
E-mail address: Salmahameed@metrohealth.org
; @SoufianAlMaha (S.T.A.)

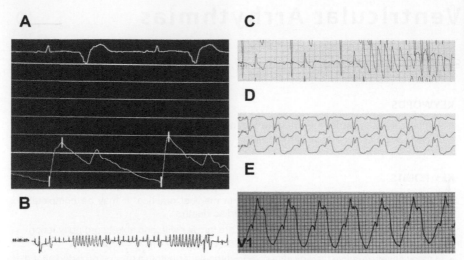

Fig. 1. (*A*) Bigeminal unifocal PVCs in patient with PVC-related cardiomyopathy. Note the low pulse pressure coincident with PVC in contrast with the normal sinus beat. (*B*) Repetitive monomorphic VT on (*A*) Holter monitor in patient with no demonstrable structural heart disease. (*C*) Unifocal bigeminal PVC initiating polymorphic VT in a patient with no demonstrable structural heart disease presenting with cardiac arrest. (*D*) Left ventricular fascicular monomorphic VT (MMVT) in patient with no demonstrable structural heart disease; note rsR in V1. (*E*) Scar-related MMVT in patient with a prior myocardial infarction; note Rsr in V1.

describes VT with a different QRS morphology among adjacent beats on the same tracing. VT is termed sustained when it is associated with hemodynamic instability or lasts for more than 30 seconds.[1,2] Repetitive MMVT refers to short bursts of non-sustained VT occurring in waves of higher frequency followed by lower frequency of occurrence (**Fig. 1**B, **Table 1**).

PATHOPHYSIOLOGY

There are 3 main mechanisms of MMVT: abnormal automaticity, triggered activity, and reentry.[3,4] Focal VT often ensues from triggered activity or abnormal automaticity (see **Table 1**). Triggered ventricular ectopy results from delayed afterdepolarization in ventricular myocytes during phase 4 of the action potential. It occurs via diastolic release of intracellular calcium and is cyclic adenosine monophosphate dependent.[5,6] In VT of triggered mechanism, each beat is a discrete event triggered by the beat before it. As such, with single PVCs, the previous sinus rhythm beat triggers the calcium release in diastole that results in the PVC. In VT, each beat of VT in turn triggers the next beat of VT. If the chain is broken, the tachycardia terminates. Repetitive MMVT is the pathognomonic form of a triggered mechanism (see **Fig. 1**B).[7] Accelerated idioventricular rhythm is the pathognomonic form of an abnormal automatic mechanism. It is often seen in the setting of reperfusion after an acute myocardial infarction.[8] Accelerated idioventricular rhythm is also observed incidentally in about 0.3% of ambulatory Holter monitors in normal adult patients. In this setting, it is typically asymptomatic and of no known clinical significance.[9]

Overwhelmingly, reentry is the most common mechanism of ventricular tachyarrhythmias. Reentrant VT occurs when a PVC encounters a heterogeneously conductive substrate within the ventricular myocardium. To initiate reentrant sustained VT, the PVC must enter the region of slow conduction in one direction but fail to conduct in

Table 1
Summary of ventricular arrhythmias based on morphology of surface electrocardiogram

Ventricular Ectopy Form	Underlying Mechanism	Clinical Significance	Treatments
Monomorphic PVC	Triggered	Benign in low burden	β-Blocker Calcium channel blocker Catheter ablation Class I AAD can be used if structurally normal heart
Multifocal PVCs	Triggered	Can be benign But often in setting of cardiomyopathy	β-Blocker Calcium channel blocker Catheter ablation often avoided
Repetitive MMVT	Triggered	Benign if low burden	β-Blocker Calcium channel blocker Catheter ablation Class I AAD can be used if structurally normal heart
Fascicular VT	Reentrant	Benign Often symptomatic	Verapamil Catheter ablation
Sustained MMVT	Reentrant usually	May present with hemodynamic compromise May signal potential for lethal VT	ICD often indicated β-Blocker Class III AAD for chronic suppression Catheter ablation
PVT	Reentrant (functional reentry)	Always malignant	ICD often indicated Treat underlying reversible causes β-Blocker

Abbreviations: AAD, antiarrhythmic drugs; ICD, implantable cardiac defibrillator.

another area of this region. Because of this unidirectional block, the impulse propagates in one direction through the region of slow conduction until it exits the other side of this region and reexcites the ventricle through the area that previously blocked. The impulse then travels through the ventricle until it finds the entrance into the region of slow conduction again, perpetuating the circuit.

MMVT in nonischemic cardiomyopathy is usually of reentrant mechanism and is mediated by idiopathic patchy intramural scar.[5,10,11] Rarely, triggered mechanisms of VT can exist in patients with nonischemic cardiomyopathy with heart failure, reduced left ventricular ejection fraction and no scar.[12]

Arrhythmogenic right ventricular dysplasia (ARVD) is a subset of nonischemic cardiomyopathy. It was once defined as the disease of the desmosomes, an intracellular junction protein that provide strong adhesion between the ventricular myocytes. Recent data have shown that ARVD pathogenesis is more complex and extends beyond desmosomal dysfunction and genetic mutations.[13] Recent data suggest a role for calcium overload in the mechanism of MMVT in early stage ARVD and hence the emerging role of flecainide drug therapy in combination with other antiarrhythmics.[14]

In contrast, PMVT results from pathologic repolarization abnormalities.[15,16] It is typically associated with significant electrolyte derangements, QT-prolonging drugs, inherited channelopathies, acute heart failure, or acute ischemia.[17] PMVT, when sustained, is equivalent to ventricular fibrillation and leads to a cardiac arrest.

The mechanism of VT in patients with no demonstrable structural heart disease is still not completely identified and thus it is called idiopathic VT. The most common regions of origin for idiopathic VT are the right ventricular and left ventricular outflow tracts (RVOT and LVOT VT). Several recent observations helped to shed more light on the pathologic basis of outflow tract VT. The inherent fiber heterogeneity in the outflow tracts, for example, has been proposed as a potential substrate for microreentry mechanisms resembling a focal site of origin. Further, some genes expressed in the atrioventricular node are expressed in the outflow tract as well and therefore increased automaticity can be seen in outflow tract cells.[18] More recently, a mutation in the SCN5A gene has been seen at a higher prevalence in patients with outflow tract PVCs, suggesting that some outflow tract ventricular arrhythmias in structurally normal hearts may represent a form of pseudo-channelopathy. Moreover, VT and PVCs in patients with no demonstrable structural heart disease may represent an early manifestation of concealed (subclinical) myopathy substrates such as ARVD, the Brugada syndrome, or catecholaminergic polymorphic VT. In such cases, it is impossible to determine the exact etiology of the VT until the syndrome manifests itself with time. Therefore, the idiopathic classification is somewhat misleading.

VENTRICULAR TACHYCARDIA ELECTROCARDIOGRAPHY

It is of paramount importance that clinicians be familiar with the different classification of ventricular arrhythmias encountered in daily practice (**Fig. 1** A–E) and acquire the electrocardiographic skills to discern VT in different clinical settings. Provided in this article is a chart from Garner and Miller,[19] who masterfully summarized the different ECG criteria, distinguishing VT from supraventricular tachycardia with aberrancy (**Fig. 2**).

CLINICAL PRESENTATION, APPROACH, AND MANAGEMENT

Idiopathic VT and PVCs most commonly originate from the RVOT, the LVOT, and the paravalvular aortic cusps. Less common sites of origin include the His-Purkinje network, the papillary muscle, the left ventricular apex, the cardiac crux, and posterior superior process of the left ventricle. Idiopathic RVOT-MMVT with a left bundle branch block and an inferior axis (positive inferior leads) on an ECG tracing represents 70% of all idiopathic VTs.[20] RVOT VT can be triggered by exercise in 25% to 50% of cases. The ECG typically shows a late precordial R wave transition. In contrast, PVCs and VT arising from the LVOT typically show an early (V2) precordial R wave transition.[21]

PVCs affect 1% of clinically normal people when screened by ECG and 40% to 75% of apparently healthy persons when screened by 24- or 48-hour Holter recordings.[22] Although in general men and women have the same incidence of PVCs on monitors, women are more likely to present with symptomatic PVCs.[23] A Swedish study of 400 men demonstrated that, regardless of the complexity of PVCs, the absence of heart disease conveyed a low risk of cardiovascular events, whereas the presence of cardiovascular disease and ventricular ectopy was associated with a cardiovascular event rate of nearly 50% after 10 years of follow-up.[24] PVCs often cause a sensation of irregular heart beat, atypical chest pain, or palpitation. Patients often describe a skipped beat. PVCs are often minimally pulsatile or nonpulsatile. Therefore, the skipped beat is often caused by the lack of pulse felt during the premature beat. The

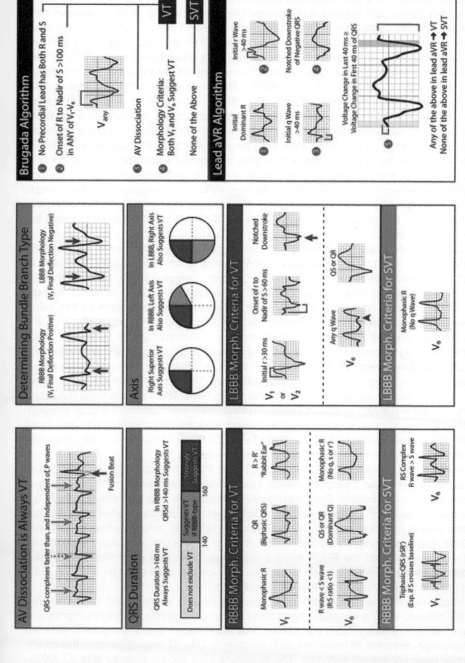

Fig. 2. The combined mechanistic and morphologic features to distinguish VT from supraventricular tachycardia with aberrancy. AV, atrioventricular; aVR, augmented vector right; LBBB, left bundle branch block; RBBB, right bundle branch block; SVT, supraventricular tachycardia. (*From* Garner JB, Miller JM. Wide Complex Tachycardia - Ventricular Tachycardia or Not Ventricular Tachycardia, That Remains the Question. Arrhythm Electrophysiol Rev 2013;2(1):25; with permission.)

following pulse, coming from the next sinus beat, is often described as a strong beat (see **Fig. 1**A).

Duffee and colleagues[25] used amiodarone to suppress frequent PVCs (>20,000/ 24 hours) in 5 patients with a cardiomyopathy without demonstrable ischemic or valvular etiology. The left ventricular function improved from 27 ± 10% to 49 ± 7% (P = .04). Bogun and colleagues retrospectively analyzed the relation between PVC burden and left ventricular systolic function in a cohort of 174 patients (57 of them with a cardiomyopathy without demonstrable ischemic or valvular etiology) who underwent radiofrequency ablation for frequent PVCs. They found that a PVC burden of 24% or greater was associated with an abnormal left ventricular systolic function at presentation (ejection fraction of ≤50%). The mean ejection fraction improved in those patients after PVC ablation from 35 ± 9% to 54 ± 10% (P = .01).[26] In current clinical practice, a PVC-related cardiomyopathy should be considered in patients with left ventricular dilatation and low systolic function in the absence of a preexisting cardiac pathology and in association with frequent PVCs. Full or partial resolution of the left ventricular systolic dysfunction after successful elimination or reduction of the PVC burden with either pharmacologic and/or catheter ablation-based therapy can be expected in such cases. Multiple studies have investigated whether certain PVC characteristics are associated with left ventricular dysfunction. PVCs with retrograde P wave, interpolated PVCs, and wider PVCs seem to be more likely to cause left ventricular dysfunction.[27,28]

Ling and colleagues[29] compared medical therapy (metoprolol, n = 50 patients and propafenone, n = 115 patients) with radiofrequency ablation for the management of PVCs originating from the RVOT in 330 patients randomized to medical therapy (n = 165 patients, mean age 50 years, 75% females) versus ablation therapy (n = 165 patients, mean age 52 years, 71% females). The outcomes of this study revealed that radiofrequency ablation of frequent idiopathic PVCs originating from the RVOT was more effective than medical therapy in decreasing the burden of PVCs and preventing recurrences. The current professional society guideline-based approach to the patient with frequent PVCs is outlined in **Fig. 3**.[30] Many patients with no structural heart disease can be treated with reassurance only. There is no role for pharmacologic or catheter ablation-based therapy in managing patients with asymptomatic PVCs and a normal left ventricular systolic function.[31] In contrast, pharmacologic and/or ablation-based therapy should be considered in patients who are very symptomatic and those with very frequent unifocal PVCs (burden of >10,000 PVCs/24 hours) with left ventricular dysfunction of potentially reversible mechanism (see **Fig. 3**).

Pharmacologic therapy for idiopathic VT and PVCs includes the use of calcium channel blockers and β-blockers, which can sometimes achieve arrhythmia suppression and symptom control. They are, however, associated with side effects and a high recurrence rate.[32,33] Catheter-based radiofrequency ablation of idiopathic VT has been proven safe and effective with a success rate that ranges between 80% and 100%. The site of origin is a major determinant of procedural success. For example, VTs originating from the RVOT have a higher success rate than those originating from the LVOT.[34] Similarly, deep intramural or epicardial sites of origin are more difficult to successfully ablate than endocardial ones.[35,36]

Idiopathic reentrant left fascicular VT, usually seen in younger and predominantly male patients with no structural heart disease, is rare and has a benign prognosis. It was first described by Zipes and colleagues.[37] Belhassen and colleagues[38] reported a very high response to treatment with verapamil. This VT originates from the inferoseptal region of the left ventricle. The signature ECG morphology for this VT (90%– 95% of cases) is of right bundle branch superior axis (see **Fig. 1**D; **Fig. 4**B). Symptoms

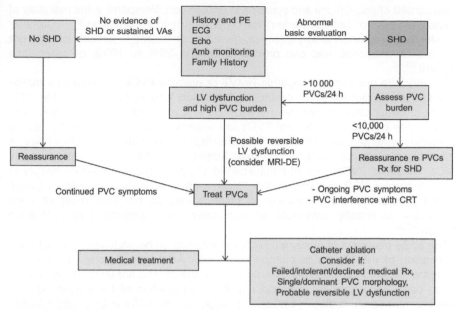

Fig. 3. Guidelines for approach and management of patients presenting with frequent unifocal PVCs. Amb, ambulatory; CRT, cardiac resynchronization therapy; LV, left ventricular; PE, physical examination; Rx, prescription; SHD, structural heart disease. (*From* Pedersen CT, Kay GN, Kalman J, et al. EHRA/HRS/APHRS Expert Consensus on Ventricular Arrhythmias. Heart Rhythm 2014;11(10):e169; with permission.)

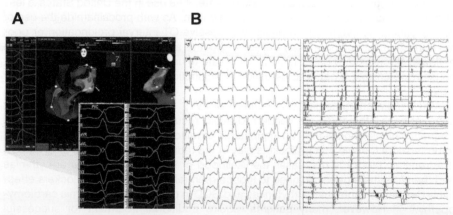

Fig. 4. (*A*) Radiofrequency ablation of unifocal PVC arising from the RVOT. The left panel is the 12-lead ECG morphology of clinical PVC mapped with early local intracardiac bipolar electrogram (*blue*) and unipolar electrogram (*yellow*). The middle panel is the 3-dimensional electroanatomic map of the RVOT in red, which signifies the endocardial site of origin of the clinical PVC. The lower panel shows excellent PVC pace mapping at site of origin. (*B*) Radiofrequency ablation of idiopathic reentrant left fascicular VT. Note the termination of VT with radiofrequency ablation targeting left posterior fascicule His-Purkinje potential (*blue arrows*).

often consist of palpitations and syncope is uncommon. Verapamil is the mainstay of medical therapy for both acute termination and chronic suppression.[39–42] Catheter radiofrequency ablation is very effective, must be considered in patients who do not respond to verapamil, and can provide a cure in 85% to 100% of cases (see **Fig. 4**B).[43–46]

On very rare occasions, idiopathic RMVT or unifocal PVCs can lead to a malignant arrhythmia like PMVT or ventricular fibrillation leading to SCD (see **Fig. 1**C). Efforts to better characterize the morphologic and electrophysiologic characteristics of these potentially malignant PVCs are underway. The role of genetic testing to identify inherited abnormalities that predispose to malignant arrhythmias is expanding. In clinical practice, high-risk features include very frequent unifocal PVCs, multifocal PVCs, runs of nonsustained VT, syncope, and a family history of SCD. A narrow QRS duration of the PVCs, with a very short coupling interval, should prompt clinical correlation in these scenarios because most of such PVCs are potentially amenable to elimination with catheter-based ablation therapy.[47,48]

The acute treatment of sustained MMVT is focused on hemodynamic stability and termination of the VT. Acute therapy starts with Advanced Cardiac Life Support guideline–directed evaluation and treatment.[49] Patients who are unstable should undergo cardiopulmonary resuscitation and have termination of the arrhythmia with direct current cardioversion.[50] Lidocaine is especially effective in terminating MMVT in the setting of acute myocardial infarction.

In patients with reentrant scar-related MMVT, procainamide has been shown to be the most effective intravenous medication for acute termination.[51,52] However, use of procainamide in this clinical setting has been limited owing to associated hypotension, a negative inotropic effect, and QT prolongation. Amiodarone is more effective than lidocaine in the treatment of acute sustained MMVT. It can be used in patients with poor renal function. However, it may take up to an hour to achieve termination of the arrhythmia with amiodarone.[53] Sotalol has been shown to be superior to lidocaine in termination of MMVT with a 69% success rate.[54] Its use in the United States is less common, although it is approved for this indication. As with procainamide the use of sotalol should be avoided with baseline excessive QT interval prolongation or poor renal function. Lidocaine is likely the least effective antiarrhythmic drug for the termination of chronic scar-related MMVT.[55] It is safe to use with renal failure and does not cause hypotension. It can also be used in conjunction with amiodarone in refractory cases.

With recurrent ischemic scar-related MMVT, suppressive pharmacologic or catheter-based therapies are needed to avoid recurrent symptoms and to prevent frequent multiple shocks from an implantable cardiac defibrillator (ICD). It is important to underscore the role that β-blockers play in the reduction of ventricular arrhythmias. β-Adrenergic blockade decreases the likelihood of triggered ventricular arrhythmias and therefore the triggers required to induce reentrant VT.[56] Use of β-blockers effectively decreases ventricular arrhythmias and SCD in patients with ischemic cardiomyopathy.[57,58] However, many patients require additional treatment for successful suppression of recurrent VT. Amiodarone is the most common antiarrhythmic drug used for suppression of the recurrent ischemic scar-related MMVT. Amiodarone reduces recurrent MMVT events more effectively than sotalol or beta-blockers. Sotalol has not been shown to reduce MMVT when compared with β-blockers, but has been shown to significantly decrease ventricular arrhythmic events compared with placebo.[59,60] However, because of the lack of long-term toxicity, in younger patients with good renal function it is often the antiarrhythmic drug of choice. The additional β-blockade can result in a significant negative inotropic effect and therefore use in the setting of poor cardiac output should be avoided.

For refractory cases of recurrent MMVT, mexiletine, an oral lidocaine analog, is used in combination with amiodarone or sotalol for ischemic scar-related MMVT suppression. However, no randomized data exist to show benefit. Class IC drugs such as flecainide or propafenone are absolutely contraindicated in this patient population based on the results of the CAST trial, where the use of flecainide and encainide resulted in increased mortality compared with placebo, owing to the proarrhythmic effects of those drugs.[61] Other antiarrhythmic drugs such as quinidine and oral procainamide have fallen out of favor owing to the potential for severe extracardiac side effects and their proarrhythmic risk. Ranolazine, a sodium channel blocker developed and used as an antianginal drug, has recently been studied as an antiarrhythmic drug. In a recent randomized trial ranolazine use in a high-risk population decreased recurrent ventricular arrhythmias requiring ICD shocks.[62]

Although advances in drug therapies in the last decade have been minimal, advances in catheter-based ablation therapy have opened new therapeutic options for patients. Catheter ablation for MMVT associated with prior myocardial infarction is focused on delivering energy into the surviving channels of ventricular myocytes that constitute the substrate for reentrant VT. These channels can be targeted by inducing the MMVT in the electrophysiology laboratory and generating an activation map of the tachycardia, thus localizing the region of slow conduction of the tachycardia and targeting this region for ablation. Alternatively, techniques have been developed for the identification of the substrate of the MMVT while in normal rhythm and targeting this substrate for ablation (**Fig. 5**). In the VANiSH trial, patients with recurrent, antiarrhythmic treated, ischemic scar-related MMVT had better outcomes with catheter ablation than with escalation of antiarrhythmic therapy.[63] More recently, a small, nonrandomized study showed that early catheter-based ablation therapy in patients with ischemic scar-related MMVT prevents recurrent ventricular arrhythmias and ICD shocks.[64] A larger prospective randomized trial is needed to assess whether catheter ablation should be offered as first-line therapy for patients presenting with sustained MMVT. Procedure-related complications occur in approximately 6% of patients, but may also depend on the severity of the underlying heart disease and other comorbidities.[65] Catheter-based ablation therapy tends to be less successful in

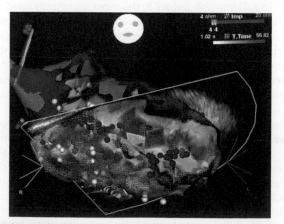

Fig. 5. Left ventricular inferior scar homogenization with radiofrequency ablation for management of reentrant scar VT in a patient with old inferior wall myocardial infarction.

patients with nonischemic scar-related MMVT with regard to both the short- and long-term VT-free survival outcomes. Ablation in patients with a nonischemic cardiomyopathy may also be more technically challenging and require epicardial access more often than in ischemic patients.[66]

It is clinically important for the internist to realize that MMVT in patients with a nonischemic cardiomyopathy should warrant further investigations, like cardiac MRI or biopsy if needed, to rule out infiltrative processes such as cardiac sarcoidosis, cardiac amyloidosis, hypertrophic cardiomyopathy, and myocarditis. This caveat has clear consequences for prognosis and management.[67] If a neuromuscular disorder is suspected, genetic testing may help to identify the underlying etiology of cardiomyopathy and give prognostic information on the potential for VT.[68] Although relatively few nonischemic patients were enrolled in trials investigating the use of ICD therapy in patients with sustained VT, most experts support the use of ICDs if no obvious reversible cause for VT is found[50]

ARVD affects 1 to 5000 of the general population with a higher prevalence in males. It is responsible for 17% of the incidence of SCD in the young in the United States. Familial ARVD accounts for 30% to 50% of cases. Several genetic mutations have been identified, the most common of which is the Plakophilin-2 (PKP2) mutation. Only 39% of affected patients have the classic fatty infiltration process limited to the right ventricle alone. Biventricular involvement is seen in about 56% of patients. Exercise is a common trigger for sustained arrhythmias and SCD in patients with ARVD.[69] Therefore, exertional palpitation or syncope, especially in the young, high-level athlete, warrants work up to exclude ARVD. The diagnosis of ARVD is complex and often difficult. It is composed of a point system that includes the patient's history, the family history, the ECG, and imaging data as outlined by the Task Force criteria for the diagnosis of ARVD.[70] Major criteria include a positive family history of confirmed ARVD in a first degree relative; precordial T wave inversion in V1-V3 or beyond in individuals greater than 14 years of age without right bundle branch block, MMVT of left bundle branch pattern and superior axis, and regional right ventricular wall motion abnormalities or aneurysm on 2-dimensional echocardiography or cardiac MRI. Not yet included in the task force criteria is the induction of VT in the electrophysiologic laboratory with a very high dose isoproterenol over 3 minutes (sensitivity >90%).[71] Syncope with exertion is also a prominent feature of ARVD.[72,73]

MMVT of a reentrant mechanism is the most common arrhythmia associated with ARVD. In addition to ICD implant, sotalol is the most commonly used first-line therapy for ARVD-VT.[74] Radiofrequency ablation is superior to medical therapy for the management of recurrent MMVT and often requires a combined endocardial–epicardial ablation approach.[75] ARVD is a progressive disease and factors that increase right ventricular wall stretch, such as exercise, are believed detrimental to its progression.[70] Patients with ARVD should not participate in competitive or endurance sports and should restrict athletic activities with the exception of low-intensity recreational sports like golf.[76]

Finally, whereas the nonsustained form of MMVT can be worked up electively, the nonsustained form of PMVT detected during outpatient cardiac monitoring is potentially a harbinger of impending cardiac arrest and must be addressed with some urgency. If seen on an outpatient monitor, it warrants immediate contact with the patient and admission to a monitored cardiac floor for inpatient workup, including a cardiology consultation and often an electrophysiology consultation. A cardiac catheterization to exclude ischemia is warranted as part of an inpatient investigation.[77] Treatment is focused on the underlying cause and evaluating for the possibility of recurrence of the arrhythmia. If the underlying cause is reversible and has been adequately addressed, then the risk of a recurrent arrhythmia is low. However, if the underlying cause cannot be reversed fully, often an ICD is used to mitigate the risk of cardiac arrest.

REFERENCES

1. Buxton AE, Lee KL, Hafley GE, et al. Limitations of ejection fraction for prediction of sudden death risk in patients with coronary artery disease: lessons from the MUSTT study. J Am Coll Cardiol 2007;50(12):1150–7.
2. Pires LA, Lehmann MH, Buxton AE, et al, Multicenter Unsustained Tachycardia Trial I. Differences in inducibility and prognosis of in-hospital versus out-of-hospital identified nonsustained ventricular tachycardia in patients with coronary artery disease: clinical and trial design implications. J Am Coll Cardiol 2001; 38(4):1156–62.
3. Wit AL, Rosen MR. Pathophysiologic mechanisms of cardiac arrhythmias. Am Heart J 1983;106(4 Pt 2):798–811.
4. Wit AL. Cellular electrophysiologic mechanisms of cardiac arrhythmias. Cardiol Clin 1990;8(3):393–409.
5. Lerman BB, Stein K, Engelstein ED, et al. Mechanism of repetitive monomorphic ventricular tachycardia. Circulation 1995;92(3):421–9.
6. Lerman BB, Ip JE, Shah BK, et al. Mechanism-specific effects of adenosine on ventricular tachycardia. J Cardiovasc Electrophysiol 2014;25(12):1350–8.
7. Enriquez A, Riley M, Marchlinski F. Noninvasive clues for diagnosing ventricular tachycardia mechanism. J Electrocardiol 2018;51(2):163–9.
8. Terkelsen CJ, Sorensen JT, Kaltoft AK, et al. Prevalence and significance of accelerated idioventricular rhythm in patients with ST-elevation myocardial infarction treated with primary percutaneous coronary intervention. Am J Cardiol 2009; 104(12):1641–6.
9. Hingorani P, Karnad DR, Rohekar P, et al. Arrhythmias seen in baseline 24-hour Holter ECG recordings in healthy normal volunteers during phase 1 clinical trials. J Clin Pharmacol 2016;56(7):885–93.
10. Josephson ME, Zimetbaum P, Huang D, et al. Pathophysiologic substrate for sustained ventricular tachycardia in coronary artery disease. Jpn Circ J 1997;61(6): 459–66.
11. Tschabrunn CM, Roujol S, Nezafat R, et al. A swine model of infarct-related reentrant ventricular tachycardia: electroanatomic, magnetic resonance, and histopathological characterization. Heart Rhythm 2016;13(1):262–73.
12. Pogwizd SM, Bers DM. Cellular basis of triggered arrhythmias in heart failure. Trends Cardiovasc Med 2004;14(2):61–6.
13. Pilichou K, Thiene G, Basso C. Assessing the significance of pathogenic mutations and autopsy findings in the light of 2010 arrhythmogenic right ventricular cardiomyopathy diagnostic criteria: a clinical challenge. Circ Cardiovasc Genet 2012;5(4):384–6.
14. Ermakov S, Gerstenfeld EP, Svetlichnaya Y, et al. Use of flecainide in combination antiarrhythmic therapy in patients with arrhythmogenic right ventricular cardiomyopathy. Heart Rhythm 2017;14(4):564–9.
15. Akar FG, Laurita KR, Rosenbaum DS. Cellular basis for dispersion of repolarization underlying reentrant arrhythmias. J Electrocardiol 2000;33(Suppl):23–31.
16. Laurita KR, Rosenbaum DS. Interdependence of modulated dispersion and tissue structure in the mechanism of unidirectional block. Circ Res 2000;87(10): 922–8.

17. Curtis MJ, Hearse DJ. Reperfusion-induced arrhythmias are critically dependent upon occluded zone size: relevance to the mechanism of arrhythmogenesis. J Mol Cell Cardiol 1989;21(6):625–37.

18. Boukens BJ, Christoffels VM, Coronel R, et al. Developmental basis for electrophysiological heterogeneity in the ventricular and outflow tract myocardium as a substrate for life-threatening ventricular arrhythmias. Circ Res 2009;104(1): 19–31.

19. B Garner J, M Miller J. Wide complex tachycardia - ventricular tachycardia or not ventricular tachycardia, that remains the question. Arrhythm Electrophysiol Rev 2013;2(1):23–9.

20. Brooks R, Burgess JH. Idiopathic ventricular tachycardia. A review. Medicine (Baltimore) 1988;67(5):271–94.

21. Betensky BP, Park RE, Marchlinski FE, et al. The V(2) transition ratio: a new electrocardiographic criterion for distinguishing left from right ventricular outflow tract tachycardia origin. J Am Coll Cardiol 2011;57(22):2255–62.

22. Kostis JB, McCrone K, Moreyra AE, et al. Premature ventricular complexes in the absence of identifiable heart disease. Circulation 1981;63(6):1351–6.

23. Sirichand S, Killu AM, Padmanabhan D, et al. Incidence of idiopathic ventricular arrhythmias: a population-based study. Circ Arrhythm Electrophysiol 2017;10(2). https://doi.org/10.1161/CIRCEP.116.004662.

24. Engstrom G, Hedblad B, Janzon L, et al. Ventricular arrhythmias during 24-h ambulatory ECG recording: incidence, risk factors and prognosis in men with and without a history of cardiovascular disease. J Intern Med 1999;246(4): 363–72.

25. Duffee DF, Shen WK, Smith HC. Suppression of frequent premature ventricular contractions and improvement of left ventricular function in patients with presumed idiopathic dilated cardiomyopathy. Mayo Clin Proc 1998;73(5):430–3.

26. Baman TS, Lange DC, Ilg KJ, et al. Relationship between burden of premature ventricular complexes and left ventricular function. Heart Rhythm 2010;7(7): 865–9.

27. Ban JE, Park HC, Park JS, et al. Electrocardiographic and electrophysiological characteristics of premature ventricular complexes associated with left ventricular dysfunction in patients without structural heart disease. Europace 2013;15(5): 735–41.

28. Del Carpio Munoz F, Syed FF, Noheria A, et al. Characteristics of premature ventricular complexes as correlates of reduced left ventricular systolic function: study of the burden, duration, coupling interval, morphology and site of origin of PVCs. J Cardiovasc Electrophysiol 2011;22(7):791–8.

29. Ling Z, Liu Z, Su L, et al. Radiofrequency ablation versus antiarrhythmic medication for treatment of ventricular premature beats from the right ventricular outflow tract: prospective randomized study. Circ Arrhythm Electrophysiol 2014;7(2): 237–43.

30. Pedersen CT, Kay GN, Kalman J, et al. EHRA/HRS/APHRS expert consensus on ventricular arrhythmias. Heart Rhythm 2014;11(10):e166–96.

31. Niwano S, Wakisaka Y, Niwano H, et al. Prognostic significance of frequent premature ventricular contractions originating from the ventricular outflow tract in patients with normal left ventricular function. Heart 2009;95(15):1230–7.

32. Buxton AE, Waxman HL, Marchlinski FE, et al. Right ventricular tachycardia: clinical and electrophysiologic characteristics. Circulation 1983;68(5):917–27.

33. Gill JS, Blaszyk K, Ward DE, et al. Verapamil for the suppression of idiopathic ventricular tachycardia of left bundle branch block-like morphology. Am Heart J 1993;126(5):1126–33.
34. Calkins H, Kalbfleisch SJ, el-Atassi R, et al. Relation between efficacy of radiofrequency catheter ablation and site of origin of idiopathic ventricular tachycardia. Am J Cardiol 1993;71(10):827–33.
35. Schweikert RA, Saliba WI, Tomassoni G, et al. Percutaneous pericardial instrumentation for endo-epicardial mapping of previously failed ablations. Circulation 2003;108(11):1329–35.
36. Rodriguez LM, Smeets JL, Timmermans C, et al. Predictors for successful ablation of right- and left-sided idiopathic ventricular tachycardia. Am J Cardiol 1997; 79(3):309–14.
37. Zipes DP, Foster PR, Troup PJ, et al. Atrial induction of ventricular tachycardia: reentry versus triggered automaticity. Am J Cardiol 1979;44(1):1–8.
38. Belhassen B, Rotmensch HH, Laniado S. Response of recurrent sustained ventricular tachycardia to verapamil. Br Heart J 1981;46(6):679–82.
39. Ohe T, Shimomura K, Aihara N, et al. Idiopathic sustained left ventricular tachycardia: clinical and electrophysiologic characteristics. Circulation 1988;77(3): 560–8.
40. German LD, Packer DL, Bardy GH, et al. Ventricular tachycardia induced by atrial stimulation in patients without symptomatic cardiac disease. Am J Cardiol 1983; 52(10):1202–7.
41. Ward DE, Nathan AW, Camm AJ. Fascicular tachycardia sensitive to calcium antagonists. Eur Heart J 1984;5(11):896–905.
42. Klein GJ, Millman PJ, Yee R. Recurrent ventricular tachycardia responsive to verapamil. Pacing Clin Electrophysiol 1984;7(6 Pt 1):938–48.
43. Wen MS, Yeh SJ, Wang CC, et al. Radiofrequency ablation therapy in idiopathic left ventricular tachycardia with no obvious structural heart disease. Circulation 1994;89(4):1690–6.
44. Nakagawa H, Beckman KJ, McClelland JH, et al. Radiofrequency catheter ablation of idiopathic left ventricular tachycardia guided by a Purkinje potential. Circulation 1993;88(6):2607–17.
45. Nogami A, Naito S, Tada H, et al. Demonstration of diastolic and presystolic Purkinje potentials as critical potentials in a macroreentry circuit of verapamil-sensitive idiopathic left ventricular tachycardia. J Am Coll Cardiol 2000;36(3): 811–23.
46. Coggins DL, Lee RJ, Sweeney J, et al. Radiofrequency catheter ablation as a cure for idiopathic tachycardia of both left and right ventricular origin. J Am Coll Cardiol 1994;23(6):1333–41.
47. Viskin S, Rosso R, Rogowski O, et al. The "short-coupled" variant of right ventricular outflow ventricular tachycardia: a not-so-benign form of benign ventricular tachycardia? J Cardiovasc Electrophysiol 2005;16(8):912–6.
48. Noda T, Shimizu W, Taguchi A, et al. Malignant entity of idiopathic ventricular fibrillation and polymorphic ventricular tachycardia initiated by premature extrasystoles originating from the right ventricular outflow tract. J Am Coll Cardiol 2005;46(7):1288–94.
49. Perkins GD, Jacobs IG, Nadkarni VM, et al. Cardiac arrest and cardiopulmonary resuscitation outcome reports: update of the Utstein Resuscitation Registry Templates for Out-of-Hospital Cardiac Arrest: a statement for healthcare professionals from a task force of the International Liaison Committee on Resuscitation (American Heart Association, European Resuscitation Council,

Australian and New Zealand Council on Resuscitation, Heart and Stroke Foundation of Canada, InterAmerican Heart Foundation, Resuscitation Council of Southern Africa, Resuscitation Council of Asia); and the American Heart Association Emergency Cardiovascular Care Committee and the Council on Cardiopulmonary, Critical Care, Perioperative and Resuscitation. Circulation 2015;132(13): 1286–300.

50. Al-Khatib SM, Stevenson WG, Ackerman MJ, et al. 2017 AHA/ACC/HRS guideline for management of patients with ventricular arrhythmias and the prevention of sudden cardiac death: executive summary: a report of the American College of Cardiology/American Heart Association Task Force on Clinical Practice Guidelines and the Heart Rhythm Society. Heart Rhythm 2018;15(10):e190–252.

51. Neumar RW, Otto CW, Link MS, et al. Part 8: adult advanced cardiovascular life support: 2010 American Heart Association Guidelines for Cardiopulmonary Resuscitation and Emergency Cardiovascular Care. Circulation 2010;122(18 Suppl 3):S729–67.

52. Gorgels AP, van den Dool A, Hofs A, et al. Comparison of procainamide and lidocaine in terminating sustained monomorphic ventricular tachycardia. Am J Cardiol 1996;78(1):43–6.

53. Tomlinson DR, Cherian P, Betts TR, et al. Intravenous amiodarone for the pharmacological termination of haemodynamically-tolerated sustained ventricular tachycardia: is bolus dose amiodarone an appropriate first-line treatment? Emerg Med J 2008;25(1):15–8.

54. Ho DS, Zecchin RP, Richards DA, et al. Double-blind trial of lignocaine versus sotalol for acute termination of spontaneous sustained ventricular tachycardia. Lancet 1994;344(8914):18–23.

55. Nasir N Jr, Taylor A, Doyle TK, et al. Evaluation of intravenous lidocaine for the termination of sustained monomorphic ventricular tachycardia in patients with coronary artery disease with or without healed myocardial infarction. Am J Cardiol 1994;74(12):1183–6.

56. Reiken S, Wehrens XH, Vest JA, et al. Beta-blockers restore calcium release channel function and improve cardiac muscle performance in human heart failure. Circulation 2003;107(19):2459–66.

57. Reiter MJ, Reiffel JA. Importance of beta blockade in the therapy of serious ventricular arrhythmias. Am J Cardiol 1998;82(4A):9I–19I.

58. Ellison KE, Hafley GE, Hickey K, et al. Effect of beta-blocking therapy on outcome in the Multicenter UnSustained Tachycardia Trial (MUSTT). Circulation 2002; 106(21):2694–9.

59. Connolly SJ, Dorian P, Roberts RS, et al. Comparison of beta-blockers, amiodarone plus beta-blockers, or sotalol for prevention of shocks from implantable cardioverter defibrillators: the OPTIC Study: a randomized trial. JAMA 2006;295(2): 165–71.

60. Pacifico A, Hohnloser SH, Williams JH, et al. Prevention of implantable-defibrillator shocks by treatment with sotalol. d,l-Sotalol Implantable Cardioverter-Defibrillator Study Group. N Engl J Med 1999;340(24):1855–62.

61. Echt DS, Liebson PR, Mitchell LB, et al. Mortality and morbidity in patients receiving encainide, flecainide, or placebo. The Cardiac Arrhythmia Suppression Trial. N Engl J Med 1991;324(12):781–8.

62. Zareba W, Daubert JP, Beck CA, et al. Ranolazine in high-risk patients with implanted cardioverter-defibrillators: the RAID trial. J Am Coll Cardiol 2018;72(6): 636–45.

63. Sapp JL, Wells GA, Parkash R, et al. Ventricular tachycardia ablation versus escalation of antiarrhythmic drugs. N Engl J Med 2016;375(2):111–21.
64. Acosta J, Cabanelas N, Penela D, et al. Long-term benefit of first-line peri-implantable cardioverter-defibrillator implant ventricular tachycardia-substrate ablation in secondary prevention patients. Europace 2017;19(6):976–82.
65. Mallidi J, Nadkarni GN, Berger RD, et al. Meta-analysis of catheter ablation as an adjunct to medical therapy for treatment of ventricular tachycardia in patients with structural heart disease. Heart Rhythm 2011;8(4):503–10.
66. Dinov B, Fiedler L, Schonbauer R, et al. Outcomes in catheter ablation of ventricular tachycardia in dilated nonischemic cardiomyopathy compared with ischemic cardiomyopathy: results from the Prospective Heart Centre of Leipzig VT (HELP-VT) Study. Circulation 2014;129(7):728–36.
67. Kuruvilla S, Adenaw N, Katwal AB, et al. Late gadolinium enhancement on cardiac magnetic resonance predicts adverse cardiovascular outcomes in nonischemic cardiomyopathy: a systematic review and meta-analysis. Circ Cardiovasc Imaging 2014;7(2):250–8.
68. Groh WJ. Arrhythmias in the muscular dystrophies. Heart Rhythm 2012;9(11): 1890–5.
69. Sawant AC, Bhonsale A, te Riele AS, et al. Exercise has a disproportionate role in the pathogenesis of arrhythmogenic right ventricular dysplasia/cardiomyopathy in patients without desmosomal mutations. J Am Heart Assoc 2014;3(6):e001471.
70. Marcus FI, McKenna WJ, Sherrill D, et al. Diagnosis of arrhythmogenic right ventricular cardiomyopathy/dysplasia: proposed modification of the task force criteria. Circulation 2010;121(13):1533–41.
71. Denis A, Sacher F, Derval N, et al. Diagnostic value of isoproterenol testing in arrhythmogenic right ventricular cardiomyopathy. Circ Arrhythm Electrophysiol 2014;7(4):590–7.
72. Wang W, Cadrin-Tourigny J, Bhonsale A, et al. Arrhythmic outcome of arrhythmogenic right ventricular cardiomyopathy patients without implantable defibrillators. J Cardiovasc Electrophysiol 2018;29(10):1396–402.
73. Dalal D, Nasir K, Bomma C, et al. Arrhythmogenic right ventricular dysplasia: a United States experience. Circulation 2005;112(25):3823–32.
74. Wichter T, Borggrefe M, Haverkamp W, et al. Efficacy of antiarrhythmic drugs in patients with arrhythmogenic right ventricular disease. Results in patients with inducible and noninducible ventricular tachycardia. Circulation 1992;86(1): 29–37.
75. Bai R, Di Biase L, Shivkumar K, et al. Ablation of ventricular arrhythmias in arrhythmogenic right ventricular dysplasia/cardiomyopathy: arrhythmia-free survival after endo-epicardial substrate based mapping and ablation. Circ Arrhythm Electrophysiol 2011;4(4):478–85.
76. Sawant AC, Te Riele AS, Tichnell C, et al. Safety of American Heart Association-recommended minimum exercise for desmosomal mutation carriers. Heart Rhythm 2016;13(1):199–207.
77. Dumas F, Cariou A, Manzo-Silberman S, et al. Immediate percutaneous coronary intervention is associated with better survival after out-of-hospital cardiac arrest: insights from the PROCAT (Parisian Region Out of hospital Cardiac ArresT) registry. Circ Cardiovasc Interv 2010;3(3):200–7.

Bradyarrhythmias for the Internist

Noha Elbanhawy, MD, MRCP, Shajil Chalil, FRCP,
Khalid Abozguia, MD, MRCP (London), PhD*

KEYWORDS

- Bradycardia • SA node • AV node • Pacemaker

KEY POINTS

- Bradycardia could be either physiologic or pathologic. The aim is always to correct any reversible cause before trying any invasive measures.
- In the acute setting, percutaneous or transvenous pacing should be considered if there is no reversible causes identified.
- Permanent pacing is the mainstay of treatment of irreversible symptomatic bradycardia or high-grade heart block even without symptoms.

INTRODUCTION

Bradycardia is defined as a sinus node rate of less than 60 beats/min. Often this can be a physiologic finding, such as in young, well-trained athletes or during sleep. It can be iatrogenic, secondary to the use of medications (**Table 1**).

Bradycardia can also occur in pathologic states as part of systemic illnesses (inflammatory-infiltrative diseases) or intrinsic cardiac conditions such as cardiomyopathies (ischemic or nonischemic), congenital heart disease, and degenerative disease of the sinoatrial (SA) node, atrioventricular (AV) node, or distal conductive system. This is in addition to cases of autonomic dysfunction with increased vagal tone or metabolic disorders (see **Table 1**).

ANATOMY OF CARDIAC CONDUCTION TISSUE
Sinoatrial Node

The SA node is a tadpole-shaped structure with a head, central body, and tail with nodal extensions representing multiple limbs. The head and proximal body portion

---

Disclosure Statement: The authors have nothing to disclose.
Lancashire Cardiac Center, Blackpool Victoria Hospital, Blackpool Teaching Hospitals Foundation Trust, Whinney Heys Road, Blackpool FY38NR, UK
* Corresponding author.
E-mail address: k.abozguia@nhs.net

Med Clin N Am 103 (2019) 897–912
https://doi.org/10.1016/j.mcna.2019.05.003
0025-7125/19/© 2019 Elsevier Inc. All rights reserved.

Table 1
Causes of bradycardias and conductive system disorders

Causes	Common Examples
Medications	1. Antihypertensives: beta blockers and calcium channel blockers 2. Antiarrhythmics: adenosine, amiodarone, dronedarone, flecainide, propafenone, and sotalol 3. Psychoactive: opioids, phenothiazines, serotonin reuptake inhibitors, tricyclic antidepressents 4. Others: digoxin, muscle relaxants, propofol
Infectious and inflammatory processes	Chagas disease, sarcoidosis, lyme disease, infective endocarditis, myocarditis
Infiltrative disorders	Amyloidosis, sarcoidosis, hemochromatosis and lymphomas
Cardiac diseases	Ischemia/infarction Cardiomyopathy (ischemic/nonischemic)
Connective tissue diseases	Rheumatoid arthritis and scleroderma
Surgical complications	Postablation or cardiac catheterization, valve surgery, and congenital heart surgery
Metabolic disorders	Acidosis, hyper- or hypokalemia, hypothermia, hypoxia, and hypothyroidism
Autonomic dysfunction	Neurocardiogenic syncope Situational syncope Carotid hypersensitivity
Others	Degenerative fibrosis and congenital heart block

of the node usually are located subepicardial beneath the fatty tissues at the junction of the superior vena cava and the right atrial appendage. It measures 8 to 22 mm long and 2 to 3 mm wide and thick.

The sinus nodes receive its blood supply through a large central artery, the sinus node artery, which is a branch of the right coronary artery in 55% to 60% of patients, and from the circumflex artery in 40% to 45%.[1,2]

Atrioventricular Node

The AV node is an interatrial structure approximately 5 mm long, 5 mm wide, and 0.8 mm thick. It is located beneath the right atrial endocardium anterior to the coronary sinus and above the insertion of the septal leaflet of the tricuspid valve. The compact node is adjacent to the central fibrous body on one side but is uninsulated by fibrous tissue on its other sides. It separates into 2 (right and left) posterior extensions toward the tricuspid and mitral annuli, respectively. The right posterior extension has been implicated as the slow pathway in typical AV nodal reentrant tachycardia.

The blood supply is predominantly from the AV nodal artery, a branch of the right coronary artery in about 90% of hearts, and from the left circumflex in 10%.

His-Purkinje System

The His bundle connects with the distal portion of the compact AV node and penetrates the central fibrous body in a leftward direction toward the crest of the interatrial septum (**Fig. 1**). It passes beneath the part of the membranous septum that adjoins the fibrous triangle between the right and noncoronary cusps. The His bundle is insulated from the atrial myocardium by the membranous septum and the ventricular myocardium by the connective tissue of the central fibrous body, thus preventing impulses from bypassing the AV node[3] (see **Fig. 1**).

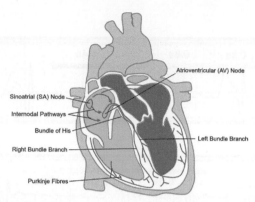

Fig. 1. Anatomy of conduction system. The conduction system of the heart. Note the SA node that is an epicardial structure commonly located at the junction between the superior vena cava and right atrium. Impulses normally conduct from the SA node down to the AV node through the atria (internodal pathways). The bundle of His then conducts impulses to the ventricles via the bundle branches and Purkinje system.

Pathologic types of bradycardia
Sinoatrial node bradycardias

Sinus bradycardia This is defined as a sinus rate less than or equal to 60 beats/min. It can be physiologic or pathologic. In general, it is mostly a benign arrhythmia, especially if the patient is asymptomatic. Iatrogenic sinus bradycardia can actually be therapeutic in patients with angina and/or heart failure where it allows for improved diastolic filling.

It can be associated with syncope, as in the cardioinhibitory response of neurocardiogenic syncope or in other pathologic states such as postmyocardial infarction (MI). When the heart rate is less than or equal to 40 beats/min and not associated with sleep or physiologic conditioning such as athletic hearts, it will often be symptomatic and patients may require consideration of permanent pacing.[4]

Sinus arrhythmia This is a phasic variation in the sinus cycle length. It is common in the young especially in those with increased vagal tone as athletes or with some drugs such as digitalis or morphine.

Respiratory form This is a normal physiologic variant commonly observed during phases of respiration. Sinus cycle length shortens during inspiration due to reflex inhibition of the vagal tone and prolongs during expiration.

Nonrespiratory form This tends to occur in older individuals with underlying cardiac disease, although sinus arrhythmia in itself is not a marker of structural heart disease. This can be difficult to distinguish from a wandering pacemaker because of variations in the P wave contour seen in the inferior leads depending on where the impulse exits the sinus node.[4]

Ventriculophasic sinus arrhythmia This is seen when sinus rhythm and heart block co-exist. The sinus cycle length (P-P interval) shortens with cycles enclosing a QRS and lengthens when there is no QRS. This might be because ventricular contraction increases the blood supply to the SA node, thus increasing its firing rate[5] (**Fig. 2D**).

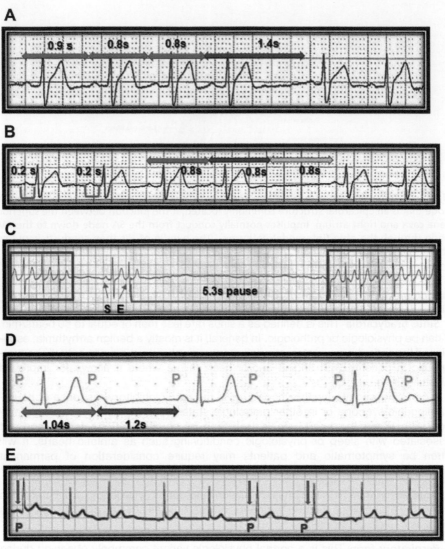

Fig. 2. SA node disease. (*A*) Type I SA exit block. Note the shortening of the P-P interval between the first and second beats. Blue arrows showing the first and second intervals, 0.9 seconds and 0.8 seconds, respectively, followed by a 1.4 second pause (*red arrow*) that is less than twice the shortest cycle length before resumption of P wave conduction. (*B*) Type II SA exit block. P-P interval, 0.8 seconds (*blue arrow*), and PR interval, 0.2 seconds, are normal and constant. The pause duration 1.6 seconds (*red and yellow arrows*) is twice the P-P interval preceding the pause. (*C*) Tachy-Brady syndrome. Atrial tachycardia (*red box*) followed by a short pause, then sinus/ectopic beats (*blue arrow*) followed by 5.3 sec pause, then resumption of tachycardia (*red box*). (*D*) Ventriculophasic sinus arrhythmia. Consecutive P waves enclosing a QRS (occur at shorter intervals than those without a QRS). (*E*) Ectopic atrial bradycardia (wandering pacemaker). Note, as the heart rate slows down, P waves become inverted with change in the PR interval indicating a shift in the dominant pacemaker site. Arrows pointing to P waves with 3 different morphologies.E, ectopic; S, sinus.

Sinus arrest (sinus pause) Sinus arrest occurs when there is complete cessation of impulse formation within the SA node. The pause will not be an exact multiple of the preceding P-P interval. Pauses up to 2 to 3 seconds can be seen in 11% of normal individuals and one-third of trained athletes. Pauses longer than 3 seconds, even if asymptomatic, are most likely related to sinus node dysfunction.[5]

Sinoatrial exit block This occurs when a normally generated impulse fails to conduct to the atrium either due to delay or due to block within the SA node or perinodal tissue. In theory, it is distinguished from a sinus pause by being an exact multiple of the preceding P-P interval. If the P-P interval is variable, such as in sinus arrhythmia, the distinction is impossible.[5]

There are 3 types of SA exit block:

- SA first-degree block is caused by prolongation of sinoatrial conduction time. It cannot be recognized on a surface electrocardiogram (ECG) and is diagnosed by invasive measurement of sinus node recording and sinoatrial conduction time in the electrophysiology (EP) laboratory.
- SA second-degree block:
  - *Type I Wenckebach* is characterized by progressive prolongation in conduction time from SA node to the atrium until there is an absent P wave. There are smaller increments in delay of impulse conduction after the initial delay, so the P-P interval tends to become shorter till a P wave fails to occur (**Fig. 2A**).
  - *Type II block* results in the absence of one or more P waves because of sudden failure of impulse exit from the sinus node resulting in pauses that should be the exact multiple of the P-P interval (**Fig. 2B**).
- SA third-degree block manifests as long pauses that cannot be distinguished from sinus arrest without invasive testing in the EP laboratory.

Isorhythmic dissociation This occurs when atrial depolarization from the sinus node or another atrial focus is slower than ventricular discharge from the AV node or bundle of His or a ventricular site, such as during an accelerated junctional rhythm.[6]

Chronotropic incompetence This is an inadequate increase in the heart rate relative to an increased metabolic demand. The resting heart rate is usually acceptable, but the patient's sinus rate does not increase as much as it should relative to the degree of activity/exercise that the patient requires. This is often a manifestation of sinus node dysfunction.[6]

Hypersensitive carotid sinus syndrome This is an abnormal response to carotid sinus massage usually related to increased vagal tone.[7] It could lead to pauses longer than 3 seconds due to sinus node exit block or arrest. An escape ventricular rhythm is usually not seen because it is suppressed by the vagal tone.

Sick sinus syndrome This is a term used to indicate a combination of SA node diseases such as sinus bradycardia, sinus pauses, and sinus exit block. All of these can occur in combination or separately (**Fig. 2A, B & C**).

Another common clinical term is tachy-brady syndrome, as patients suffer from periods of sinus bradycardia alternating with periods of atrial tachyarrhythmias such as atrial fibrillation, atrial flutter, and atrial tachycardias. Patients also tend to have long "conversion" pauses when converting from the tachycardia into sinus rhythm. Many of these patients will benefit from permanent pacemakers, as this will enable safe use of antiarrhythmic medications or rate-controlling AV nodal blockers to treat the intermittent tachycardias.

Other Types of Atrial Bradyarrhythmias

Ectopic atrial bradycardia (wandering pacemaker)

The dominant pacemaker is a focus firing with a higher automaticity than the sinus node usually in the lower crista terminalis or the AV junction. If more than 3 P waves are seen, then the rhythm is named a "wandering atrial pacemaker." The ECG shows variation in the RR interval. The PR can shorten and become less than 120 ms, and the P wave can change in contour to become negative in leads I and II or disappear into the QRS (**Fig. 2**E). This is often normal in young individuals or athletes.

Bradycardias due to atrioventricular nodal disease

First-degree atrioventricular nodal heart block Every atrial impulse is conducted to the ventricles but with a prolonged PR that is fixed. It is longer than 0.2 seconds but could be as long as 1.0 seconds. Prolongation usually results from conduction delay in the AV node.

Second-degree atrioventricular nodal heart block There is intermittent failure of conduction of an atrial impulse to the ventricle. The conduction failure can be at the level of the AV node or in the His–Purkinje system (HPS). Intracardiac recordings are the most accurate in localizing the site of block. However, a narrow QRS typically indicates block at the level of the AV node, whereas a wide QRS in the HPS. If more than one P wave is consecutively not conducted, the block is either high degree or complete. There are 2 types of second-degree AV block:

- *Mobitz type I (Wenckebach)*: this is typically more benign, less likely to give symptoms and to progress to higher degree block. However, the elderly might be more symptomatic by virtue of fatigue, lightheadedness, or near syncope. In this type of block there is progressive prolongation of the PR interval until failure of conduction occurs. On a surface ECG, it is recognized by the progressive prolongation of the PR interval followed by a nonconducted P wave. The PR interval following this pause is shorter than the PR interval before the block. The QRS is typically narrow (**Fig. 3**A).
- *Mobitz type II*: this type of block is characterized on the surface ECG by a sudden failure of P wave conduction to the ventricles, without progressive prolongation of the PR interval. The P-P interval remains constant, and the pause following the block is usually twice the P-P interval. The QRS is typically wide (**Fig. 3**B).

Second-degree 2:1 heart block In this case, atrial impulses are conducted with a 2:1 ratio. The PR interval is constant, provided the rhythm is regular. Because the nonconducted P wave occurs every other beat, one cannot distinguish between type 1 and 2 blocks (**Fig. 3**C). Some of the features that help localize the site of block include the following:

1. A narrow QRS favors type 1 AV nodal block, whereas a wide QRS favors type 2 infranodal disease.
2. Fixed 2:1 block with PR less than 160 ms suggests infranodal block but long PR greater than 300 ms suggests AV nodal block.
3. Presence of Wenckebach before or after the presence of 2:1 block indicates AV nodal block.
4. Improvement with atropine or exercise suggests AV nodal block.

Third-degree atrioventricular nodal heart block This is a complete failure of conduction of impulses from the atrium to the ventricles. The block could be at the level

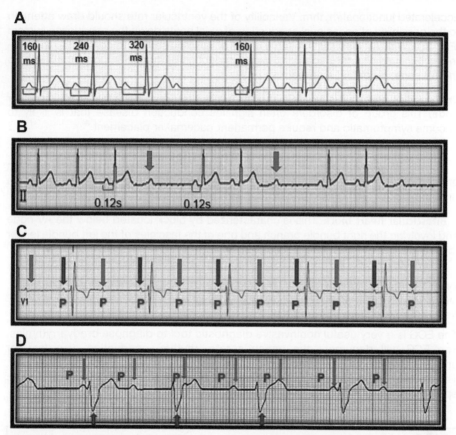

Fig. 3. AV node disease. (*A*) Mobitz type I second-degree heart block. There is progressive prolongation of PR interval before failure of conduction to the ventricle. The PR following the block is shorter than PR interval before the block. (*B*) Mobitz type 2 second-degree heart block. ECG showing normal PR with 1:1 conduction followed by block without any prolongation of the PR interval. Blue arrows showing nonconducted P waves. (*C*) 2:1 Heart block. A 2:1 pattern with normal PR for the conducted beats. Blue arrows point to nonconducted P waves. Red arrows point to conducted P waves.(*D*) Complete heart block. There is no fixed relationship between the atrial (*blue arrows*) and ventricular escape beats (*red arrows*).

of the AV node or the HPS. Escape rhythms usually arise just distal to the site of block. In case of block at the level of the AV node, the junctional escape is usually at a rate of 40 to 50 beats/min. Block in the HPS is usually associated with slower escape rhythms with rates less than 40 b/min.

Block at the level of the AV node is common in patients with congenital heart block or in cases that are transient such as those secondary to drugs (ie, digitalis, beta blockers, and calcium channel blockers) or following inferior MIs. The AV node will typically recover and respond to atropine, unlike the block in the distal HPS. Although not always clear on a surface ECG, intracardiac recordings easily show the level of block whether supra, intra or infrahisian.[8]

Atrioventricular dissociation AV dissociation is a form of complete heart block that occurs when the atrial rate is slower than the ventricular rate as in the case of an accelerated junctional rhythm. Variability of the ventricular rate should draw attention to the possibility of occasional conduction of atrial beats down the conduction system (**Fig. 3**D). With AV dissociation some of the atrial impulses fail to conduct to the ventricles because of retrograde concealed conduction of the faster junctional beats up the AV node, rendering it refractory.

Bradycardias due to His-Purkinje system tissue disease (below the atrioventricular node) This group of disorders often signifies conduction disease that is likely to become symptomatic and require permanent pacemaker placement.[6]
Common features and types of bundle branch block are described in **Table 2**.

Nonspecific intraventricular conduction delay This is defined as QRS duration greater than 100 and less than 120 ms, where morphology criteria for right bundle branch block or left bundle branch block are not present.

Bifascicular heart block This is characterized by block located below the AV node and involving the right bundle branch and one of the fascicles of the left bundle (either the left anterior or left posterior fascicle).[9]

INVESTIGATIONS IN PATIENTS WITH SUSPECTED OR DOCUMENTED BRADYCARDIA OR CONDUCTION DISORDERS
Resting 12-Lead Electrocardiogram

The ECG is a very useful noninvasive diagnostic tool to diagnose bradyarrythmias. The ECG will document the patient's rate, rhythm, conduction disorders, or any signs that suggest structural heart disease or electrolyte disturbances. The highest yield for an ECG is when it is recorded during a symptomatic episode.[10,11]

Table 2
Characteristics and types of bundle branch block

Complete RBBB	Complete LBBB
QRS duration ≥120 ms	QRS duration ≥120 ms
V1 Positive rSR′ (Rabbit Ear) R′ wider than the initial R wave	V1 negative (rS pattern)
V6 Positive QRS S wave duration > R	V6 Positive and notched (R pattern) ST and T wave change in opposite direction to QRS

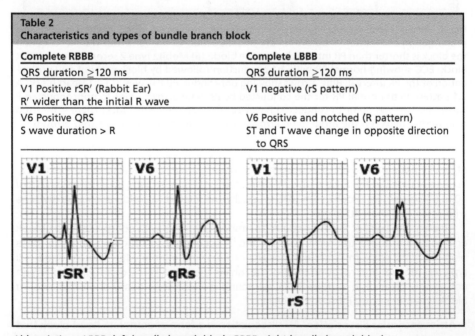

Abbreviations: LBBB, left bundle branch block; RBBB, right bundle branch block.

Exercise Electrocardiographic Testing

This is not routinely done for patients with suspected bradycardia but can be useful in a select group with possible sinus node chronotropic incompetence or exercise-induced AV block. Sinus node incompetence is usually demonstrated by a failure to increase the heart rate beyond 80% during peak exercise with associated symptoms as presyncope or syncope.[12–16] Exercise can help uncover the level of block in patients with second- or third-degree heart block. With increased sympathetic tone and vagal inhibition, the sinus rate increases. If the level of block is at the AV node, then cardiac conduction will improve and the ventricular rate will also increase. If the level of block is below the AV node, higher degree of block will develop as the HPS becomes refractory.

Ambulatory Electrocardiogram

Other articles in this issue will cover the many means of externally monitoring the rhythm and establishing a clear symptom/rhythm correlation. They are selected based on the frequency of the symptoms. They can be as short as 24-hour Holter monitors[17–19] or as long as 4-week event monitors. Emerging newer technology based on smartphone applications is being used more frequently to establish symptoms/rhythm correlation.

Imaging

Transthoracic echocardiograms (TTEs) are an important noninvasive and easily applicable tool to assess for structural heart disease and different forms of cardiomyopathies in patients with bradycardia. An assessment of the left ventricular function is often paramount in considering the type of device needed in patients with bradyarrhythmias. When a TTE quality is not optimal, other imaging modalities including transoesophageal echocardiogram, cardiac magnetic resonance imaging, computed tomography, and nuclear imaging (PET scans) can be useful.[20,21]

Laboratory Testing

Blood laboratory tests are routinely performed in patients with bradyarrhythmia. These tests provide information about potential underlying systemic illness that can contribute to bradycardia. These include thyroid function testing, Lyme titer in endemic areas, potassium levels, and the PH balance.[22,23]

Genetic Testing and Counseling

These tests are not routinely done but are helpful in selected patients with suspected hereditary conduction disease, patients with isolated conduction disease, or those with congenital heart disease.

Cardiac conduction diseases could precede the development of a dilated cardiomyopathy, such as in the laminopathies (LMNA gene). The cardiac involvement in laminopathies usually presents with progressive atrioventricular block, followed by a dilated cardiomyopathy, sudden cardiac death, and more infrequently, atrial arrhythmias.[24,25]

Sleep Apnea Studies (Polysomnography)

Polysomnography is useful in patients with suspected obstructive sleep apnea who frequently have nocturnal bradyarrhythmias and heart block. Treatment with continuous positive airway pressure has been found to reduce sleep-related bradyarrhythmias significantly.[26] These patients often will not require pacing.

Invasive Testing

Implantable loop recorders

Implantable loop recorders (ILRs) are subcutaneous devices implanted just left of the sternum, over the heart, with a battery life that can last for up to 3 years. They are most useful in patients with infrequent symptoms of palpitation, near syncope or syncope (eg,>30 days) and where it is challenging to provide clear symptom/rhythm correlation. These devices have the capability of autorecording electrograms based on a preset of programmed parameters in addition to events triggered by patients.[27,28]

Electrophysiologic studies

EP studies are invasive tests and usually indicated in patients with suspected conduction disease but no clear symptom/rhythm correlation despite extensive noninvasive testing. Sinus node and AV node functions are tested, and pharmacologic provocation with several drugs including atropine, isoprenaline, and procainamide can be used to uncover pathology in the cardiac conduction system (**Fig. 4** and **Table 3**).[29–31]

PRINCIPLES OF MANAGEMENT

In patients with severe bradycardia, some general measures include correcting electrolyte imbalances, withdrawing offending drugs such as beta blockers, calcium

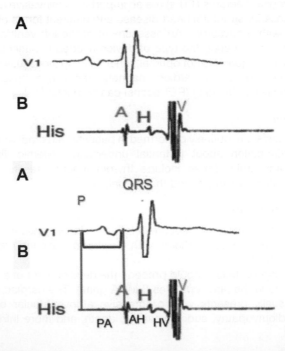

Fig. 4. Baseline intervals. (*A*) A surface ECG. PR interval represents conduction from the atrium across the AV node to the ventricle to generate a QRS. (*B*) Corresponding intracardiac His recording. PA interval from surface P to intracardiac His A represents conduction from a fixed point in the atrium, usually SA node to the AV node region. AH represents conduction from atrium to the His bundle and HV represents distal conduction from the His to the ventricle. *Top panel* without interval labeling. *Bottom panel* with interval and labeling.

Table 3 Baseline intervals			
	PA	**AH**	**HV**
Baseline Interval	Earliest recorded atrial activity on any channel and rapid deflection of atrial electrogram on His bundle catheter Prolonged if diseased atrium or drugs	From atrial electrogram at His bundle catheter to beginning of His deflection. Prolonged with AV node disease or autonomic tone or drugs	From His electrogram to earliest ventricular activation. Prolonged with His-Purkinje system disease
Specific measurement	25–55 ms	55–125 ms	35–55 ms

channel blockers, or ivabradine, and treating infections such as lyme disease or underlying myocardial ischemia. Whenever sinus node dysfunction is seen; it is important to identify and treat underlying reversible conditions such as hypothyroidism, hypoxia, and hypervagotonia.

Drugs such as atropine, epinephrine, and isoprenaline can be used to either temporarily increase the underlying heart rate or reverse the effects of certain medications.

Percutaneous or transvenous temporary pacing should be considered in the acute setting when patients are highly symptomatic or unstable. With percutaneous pacing, sedation is needed and ensuring an adequate output and capture of myocardium with a good peripheral pulse is crucial. When needed, transvenous pacing can be a useful bridge to permanent pacing. However, it can be associated with complications such as cardiac perforation, tamponade, pneumothorax, infection, and lead displacement.

Permanent Pacing

Regardless of the level of heart block, permanent pacing should be considered in all patients with symptomatic bradycardia and without identifiable reversible causes. In patients with second- or third-degree AV block, permanent pacing should be considered in asymptomatic patients, especially if their heart rates are less than 40 b/min or if they have pauses longer than 3 seconds (Class I recommendation). Patients with atrial fibrillation with one or more pauses more than 5 seconds need pacing even if asymptomatic (Class I recommendation).

Temporary heart block is commonly seen in patients with acute MIs or patients undergoing coronary revascularization. This usually resolves in the setting of inferior MIs. If seen in anterior MIs, this often indicates extensive myocardial damage. If heart block persists (more likely with anterior MI), permanent pacing is usually indicated.[32]

Pacing Modes (Pacemaker Nomenclature)

Permanent pacemakers are either single (such as AAI or VVI) or dual chamber (DDD) pacemaker:

- The first letter refers to the chamber paced.
- The second letter refers to the chamber sensed.
- The third letter refers to the response to a sensed event. This can be inhibition (I) of activity or triggering (T) of activity or both (D). For example, in a DDD pacemaker, a sensed P wave inhibits the atrial lead but triggers the ventricular lead to pace after a programmed delay (AV delay).

- Biventricular pacing (also referred to as chronic resynchronization therapy or CRT) refers to the presence of an additional left ventricular lead inserted in a branch of the coronary sinus. It could be programmed either in VVI mode (if no atrial lead is present, ie, patients with atrial fibrillation) or in DDD mode (with an atrial lead for synchronous AV pacing)[33] (**Table 4**).

Rate response(R)

Rate response(R) is a feature present in all modern day devices, single or dual chamber. The pacing rate is increased based on sensors in the pacemaker generator that can detect motion, minute ventilation, or changes in thoracic impedence. If this feature is enabled, then it will usually be added as fourth letter such as DDD(R) or VVI(R).

VVI(R)

Single ventricular lead pacing is reserved today for patients in whom atrial pacing and sensing are not necessary, such as in patients with permanent atrial fibrillation or those with multiple comorbidities and poor activity levels where single chamber pacing provides similar benefit to dual chamber pacing without the risks of adding a lead placement. VVI pacing is also indicated in patients with atrial standstill where the atrium cannot be paced.

VDD(R)

This device is a single ventricular lead device with an atrial bipole used to sense atrial activity. It can only pace the ventricle. It can maintain AV synchrony and rate response especially in young patients without the need for added atrial pacing lead.

DDD(R)

This is by far the most common device placed today. It has 2 leads implanted in the atrium and ventricle for sensing and pacing both chambers. It is the preferred modality in patients with sinus node dysfunction and AV block. It maintains AV synchrony and rate responsiveness over a wide variety of pathologies. In addition, the atrial lead can detect atrial tachyarrhythmias and mode switch accordingly to VVI pacing so not to track atrial tachyarrhythmias.

AAI(R)

Single atrial lead pacing can be used in patients with isolated sinus node dysfunction, although currently DDD pacing is the preferred modality because some patients will eventually develop AV block.

DDD—cardiac synchronization therapy pacemaker (biventricular pacing)

This device is a dual chamber pacemaker with an added left ventricular lead. It is used to resynchronize the right ventricle and left ventricle and is indicated in patients with clinically significant symptomatic heart failure (NYHA class II–IV, ejection fraction <35%) with wide QRS complexes (>150 ms) and evidence of ventricular dyssynchrony (left bundle branch block).

Leadless pacemakers

More recently, leadless pacing has been developed to avoid the complications associated with an indwelling endovascular lead and subcutaneous generator pocket. It was first introduced in the 1970s but only became commercially available in the last decade. It is a dime-sized capsule implanted directly into the right ventricular apex using a delivery system through the right femoral vein. Currently available are the Nanostim leadless pacemaker (St. Jude Medical, St. Paul, MN, USA) and the Micra Transcatheter Pacing System (Medtronic, Minneapolis, MN, USA). These devices

Table 4						
Pacing modes						
Pacing Mode	VVI	AAI	VDD	DDD	Leadless	CRT-P
Leads	Single	Single	Single With sensor at proximal atrial end	Atrial and ventricular	Small device implanted in the RV apex (no leads)	Right atrium, right ventricle, and left ventricle via coronary sinus
Sensing	Ventricle	Atrium	Both chamber	Both chambers	Ventricle only	Right atrium and right ventricle
Pacing	Ventricle	Atrium	Ventricle Only	Both chambers	Ventricle only	Right atrium, right and left ventricles
Indication	If atrial pacing not required or possible, for example, AF or debilitated elderly patients	Isolated sinus node disease with intact AV node conduction (rarely used nowadays)	AV node disease with intact SA node—maintains AV synchrony	Most commonly used with both SA node and AV node disease to maintain AV synchrony	Same as VVI	Patients with symptomatic heart failure with severe LV systolic dysfunction, LBBB pattern, and wide QRS>150 ms

significantly reduce the risks related to an endovascular pacing lead and a subcutaneous pocket, such as vascular occlusion, tricuspid insufficiency, and endovascular infections including endocarditis.[34,35]

SUMMARY

Bradycardia could be either physiologic or pathologic. The aim is always to correct any reversible cause before trying any invasive measures. In the acute setting, percutaneous or transvenous pacing should be considered if there is no reversible causes identified. Permanent pacing is the mainstay of treatment of irreversible symptomatic bradycardia or high-grade heart block even without symptoms.

ACKNOWLEDGMENTS

We would to thank Dr Dinesh Kumar Srinivasan (Associate Professor, Yong Loo Lin School of Medicine, National University of Singapore, Singapore) for his assistance in **Fig. 1**.

REFERENCES

1. Murphy C, Lazzara R. Current concepts of anatomy and electrophysiology of the sinus node. J Interv Card Electrophysiol 2016;46:9–18.
2. Ho SY, Sánchez-Quintana D. Anatomy and pathology of the sinus node. J Interv Card Electrophysiol 2016;46:3–8.
3. Dandamudi G, Vijayaraman P. The complexity of the His bundle: understanding its anatomy and physiology through the lens of the past and the present. Pacing-ClinElectrophysiol 2016;39:1294–7.
4. Zipes DP, Libby P, Bonow RO, et al. Bradyarrhythmias and Atrioventricular block. In: Bonow RO, Mann DL, Tomaselli GF, editors. Braunwald's heart disease: a textbook of cardiovascular medicine, single volume. 11th edition. Philadelphia: Elseiver/Saunders; 2018. p. 772–9.
5. Issa ZF, Miller JM, Zipes DP. Sinus node dysfunction. In: Olgin JE, Zipes DP, editors. Clinical arrhythmology and electrophysiology: a companion to Braunwald's heart disease. 3rd edition. Philadelphia: Elsevier/Saunders; 2019. p. 238–54.
6. Writing Committee Members, Kusumoto FM, Schoenfeld MH, Barrett C. 2018 ACC/AHA/HRS Guideline on the evaluation and management of patients with bradycardia and cardiac conduction delay: A Report of the American College of Cardiology/American Heart Association Task Force on Clinical Practice Guidelines and the Heart Rhythm Society. Heart Rhythm 2018. https://doi.org/10.1016/j.hrthm.2018.10.037.
7. Sheldon RS, Grubb BP 2nd, Olshansky B, et al. Heart Rhythm Society expert consensus statement on the diagnosis and treatment of postural tachycardia syndrome, inappropriate sinus tachycardia, and vasovagal syncope. Heart Rhythm 2015;12:e41–63.
8. Nelson WP. Diagnostic and prognostic implications of surface recordings from patients with atrioventricular block. Card ElectrophysiolClin 2016;8:25–35.
9. Glenn N. Levine cardiac pacing for bradycardia, heart block and heart failure. In: Levine GN, editor. Cardiology secrets. 5th edition. Philadelphia: Elseiver/Saunders; 2018. p. 344–51.
10. Linzer M, Yang EH, Estes NA 3rd, et al. Diagnosing syncope. Part 1: value of history, physical examination, and electrocardiography. Clinical efficacy

Assessment Project of the American College of Physicians. Ann Intern Med 1997; 126:989–96.

11. Perez-Rodon J, Martinez-Alday J, Baron-Esquivias G, et al. Prognostic value of the electrocardiogram in patients with syncope: data from the group for syncope study in the emergency room (GESINUR). Heart Rhythm 2014;11:2035–44.

12. Savonen KP, Kiviniemi V, Laukkanen JA, et al. Chronotropic incompetence and mortality in middle-aged men with known or suspected coronary heart disease. EurHeart J 2008;29:1896–902.

13. Miller J, Issa Z. Atrioventricular conduction abnormalities. In: Issa ZF, Miller JM, Zipes DP, editors. Clinical arrhythmology and electrophysiology: a companion to Braunwald's heart disease. 3rd edition. Philadelphia: Elseiver/Saunders; 2019. p. 255–85.

14. Coplan NL, Morales MC, Romanello P, et al. Exercise-related atrioventricular block. Influence of myocardial ischemia. Chest 1991;100:1728–30.

15. Oliveros RA, Seaworth J, Weiland FL, et al. Intermittent left anterior hemiblock during treadmill exercise test. Correlation with coronary arteriogram. Chest 1977;72:492–4.

16. AlJaroudi WA, Alraies MC, Wazni O, et al. Yield and diagnostic value of stress myocardial perfusion imaging in patients without known coronary artery disease presenting with syncope. CircCardiovascImaging 2013;6:384–91.

17. Barrett PM, Komatireddy R, Haaser S, et al. Comparison of 24-hour Holter monitoring with 14-day novel adhesive patch electrocardiographic monitoring. Am J Med 2014;127:95.e11-7.

18. Joshi AK, Kowey PR, Prystowsky EN, et al. First experience with a mobile cardiac outpatient telemetry (MCOT) system for the diagnosis and management of cardiac arrhythmia. Am J Cardiol 2005;95:878–81.

19. Steinberg JS, Varma N, Cygankiewicz I, et al. 2017 ISHNE-HRS expert consensus statement on ambulatory ECG and external cardiac monitoring/telemetry. Heart Rhythm 2017;14:e55–96.

20. Douglas PS, Garcia MJ, Haines DE, et al. ACCF/ASE/AHA/ASNC/HFSA/HRS/SCAI/SCCM/SCCT/SCMR 2011 appropriate use criteria for echocardiography. J Am SocEchocardiogr 2011;24(3):229–67.

21. Hendel RC, Patel MR, Kramer CM, et al. ACCF/ACR/SCCT/SCMR/ASNC/NASCI/SCAI/SIR 2006 appropriateness criteria for cardiac computed tomography and cardiac magnetic resonance imaging. J Am CollRadiol 2006;3(10):751–71.

22. Chon SB, Kwak YH, Hwang SS, et al. Severe hyperkalemia can be detected immediately by quantitative electrocardiography and clinical history in patients with symptomatic or extreme bradycardia: a retrospective cross-sectional study. J CritCare 2013;28:1112.e7-13.

23. Wan D, Blakely C, Branscombe P, et al. Lyme carditis and high-degree atrioventricular block. Am J Cardiol 2018;121:1102–4.

24. Pan H, Richards AA, Zhu X, et al. A novel mutation in *LAMIN A/C* is associated with isolated early-onset atrial fibrillation and progressive atrioventricular block followed by cardiomyopathy and sudden cardiac death. Heart Rhythm 2009. https://doi.org/10.1016/j.hrthm.2009.01.037.

25. Ishikawa T, Tsuji Y, Makita N. Inherited bradyarrhythmia: a diverse genetic background. J Arrhythm 2016;32:352–8.

26. Kasai T, Floras JS, Bradley TD. Sleep apnea and cardiovascular disease: a bidirectional relationship. Circulation 2012;126:1495–510.

27. Shen WK, Sheldon RS, Benditt DG, et al. 2017 ACC/AHA/HRS guideline for the evaluation and management of patients with syncope: a report of the American

College of Cardiology/American Heart Association Task Force on Clinical Practice Guidelines and the Heart Rhythm Society. J Am CollCardiol 2017;70: e39–110.

28. Podoleanu C, DaCosta A, Defaye P, et al. Early use of an implantable loop recorder in syncope evaluation: a randomized study in the context of the French healthcare system (FRESH study). Arch Cardiovasc Dis 2014;107:546–52.

29. Krol RB, Morady F, Flaker GC, et al. Electrophysiologic testing in patients with unexplained syncope: Clinical and noninvasive predictors of outcome. J Am CollCardiol 1987;10:358–63.

30. Denniss AR, Ross DL, Richards DA, et al. Electrophysiologic studies in patients with unexplained syncope. Int J Cardiol 1992;35:211–7.

31. Graff B, Graff G, Koźluk E, et al. Electrophysiological features in patients with sinus node dysfunction and vasovagal syncope. Arch Med Sci 2011;7:963–70.

32. Epstein AE, DiMarco JP, Ellenbogen KA, et al. 2012 ACCF/AHA/HRS focused update incorporated into the ACCF/AHA/HRS 2008 guidelines for device-based therapy of cardiac rhythm abnormalities: a report of the American College of Cardiology Foundation/American Heart Association Task Force on Practice Guide. Circulation 2013;127:e283–352.

33. Gillis AM, Russo AM, Ellenbogen KA, et al. HRS/ACCF expert consensus statement on pacemaker device and mode selection. J Am CollCardiol 2012;60: 682–703.

34. Kusumoto FM, Schoenfeld MH, Wilkoff BL, et al. 2017 HRS Expert consensus statement on cardiovascular implantable electronic device lead management and extraction. Heart Rhythm 2017;14:e503–51.

35. Tjong FVY, Knops RE, Udo EO, et al. Leadless pacemaker versus transvenous single-chamber pacemaker therapy: a propensity score-matched analysis. Heart Rhythm 2018;15:1387–93.

Sudden Cardiac Death
Who Is at Risk?

Mohammad-Ali Jazayeri, MD[a], Martin P. Emert, MD, FHRS[b],*

KEYWORDS

- Sudden cardiac death • Cardiac arrest • Electrophysiology
- Implantable cardioverter-defibrillator • Arrhythmias • Ventricular tachycardia
- Ventricular fibrillation • Ischemic heart disease

KEY POINTS

- Sudden cardiac death (SCD) is the number 1 killer in America.
- Half of SCD events occurring in patients with coronary disease represent the first manifestation of their cardiovascular disease, and a large proportion of SCD occurs in those not known to be at risk.
- Patients with a left ventricular ejection fraction less than or equal to 35%, regardless of whether they have ischemic or nonischemic cardiomyopathy, are at high risk for SCD and should be evaluated for an implantable cardioverter-defibrillator (ICD).
- In high-risk populations, SCD can be prevented with an ICD, a lifesaving and cost-effective intervention in appropriate candidates.
- The number of annual SCD events remains unacceptably high and underscores the need for better risk assessment tools to guide therapy.

INTRODUCTION

Sudden cardiac death (SCD) is a leading cause of death in the United States and is estimated to be responsible for 170,000 to 450,000 deaths annually.[1] Mortality from SCD exceeds the combined mortality of all major cancers (lung, breast, colorectal, and prostate).[2] Preexisting heart disease is present in nearly 80% of patients with SCD.[3,4] In the coronary heart disease (CHD) population, 50% of SCD events represent the first clinical manifestation of cardiovascular disease.[5] Deaths due to CHD have decreased in recent decades owing to effective therapies for its management and prevention.[6] Despite the parallel reduction in the absolute incidence of SCD over the past 50 years,[4,6,7] the incidence of SCD as a proportion of overall cardiovascular death

Disclosure Statement: Neither of the authors has any relevant conflict of interest to report.
[a] Department of Cardiovascular Medicine, University of Kansas Medical Center, 3901 Rainbow Boulevard, Mailstop 3006, Kansas City, KS 66160, USA; [b] Division of Electrophysiology, Department of Cardiology, University of Kansas Medical Center, 4000 Cambridge Street, Mailstop 4023, Kansas City, KS 66160, USA
* Corresponding author.
E-mail address: mpemert@kumc.edu

remains relatively unchanged at around 50%.[8,9] These observations raise the question, "Who is at risk for SCD?" This article aims to answer this question and, in the process, review the definition, pathophysiology, epidemiology, and risk factors of SCD, followed by a discussion on the evaluation of patients at risk for SCD and appropriate treatment strategies.

DEFINITION OF SUDDEN CARDIAC DEATH

SCD is defined as "sudden and unexpected death occurring within an hour of the onset of symptoms, or occurring in patients found dead within 24 hours of being asymptomatic and presumably due to a cardiac arrhythmia or hemodynamic catastrophe."[1,10] SCD is to be differentiated from sudden cardiac arrest (SCA), which, unlike SCD, is not fatal. If attempts to restore circulation are unsuccessful in SCA, this is referred to as SCD.[10,11] Underlying arrhythmias are thought to be the mechanism of death in SCD. In patients undergoing ambulatory electrocardiographic monitoring at the time of SCD, ventricular tachycardia (VT) and ventricular fibrillation (VF) made up approximately 85% of SCD events, whereas bradyarrhythmias accounted for the remaining 15%.[12]

PATHOPHYSIOLOGY OF SUDDEN CARDIAC DEATH

The conditions associated with SCD are heterogeneous (**Box 1**). The pathophysiology of SCD involves a complex interplay of factors, broadly categorized as structural, functional, and electrogenic, all associated with SCD (**Fig. 1**). It is postulated that for an electrogenic event, such as a premature ventricular contraction (PVC), to cause a cardiac arrest, there must be a substrate (structural element) present; for example, prior myocardial infarction (MI), hypertrophy, or cardiomyopathy. This substrate is then modulated by a trigger (functional phenomena); for example, hemodynamic instability, ischemia, or electrolyte abnormalities, which together may result in an ordinarily benign PVC causing a fatal VT or VF episode (SCD).[13] However, not all conditions associated with SCD are primarily cardiac in origin; several are noncardiac entities (see **Box 1**).

Box 1
Major conditions associated with sudden cardiac death

Ischemic heart disease
    Coronary artery disease (CAD) with MI or angina
    Coronary artery embolism
    Nonatherogenic CAD (arteritis, dissection, and congenital coronary anomalies)
    Coronary artery spasm

Nonischemic heart disease
    Hypertrophic cardiomyopathy
    Dilated cardiomyopathy
    Valvular heart disease
    Congenital heart disease
    Arrhythmogenic right ventricular cardiomyopathy
    Myocarditis
    Cardiac sarcoidosis
    Cardiac tamponade
    Acute myocardial rupture
    Aortic dissection
    Neuromuscular disorders (eg, Duchenne, Becker, and Emery-Dreifuss muscular dystrophies)

Structurally normal heart or primary electrophysiological conditions
 Idiopathic VF or J-wave syndrome
 Brugada syndrome
 Long QT syndrome
 Short QT syndrome
 Catecholaminergic polymorphic MI
 Preexcitation syndrome
 High-grade atrioventricular block with torsades de pointes
 Familial SCD
 Commotio cordis

Noncardiac diseases
 Pulmonary embolism
 Intracranial hemorrhage
 Drowning
 Pickwickian syndrome
 Drug overdose or toxicity
 Central airway obstruction
 Sudden infant death syndrome

EPIDEMIOLOGY OF SUDDEN CARDIAC DEATH

SCD has a reported incidence of approximately 0.1% to 0.2% per year and is estimated to cause 170,000 to 450,000 deaths annually, depending on the reporting method used.[1] Furthermore, the estimated occurrence of premature death in US men and women was greater for SCD than all individual cancers and most other major causes of death,[2] accounting for up to 18% of all deaths in the United States.[2,14] From the cardiovascular perspective, up to 50% of all cardiac deaths are due to SCD.[8] A key principle in understanding why, despite numerous medical and technological advances, the public health burden of SCD remains high is illustrated in **Fig. 2**. Although the overall incidence of SCD

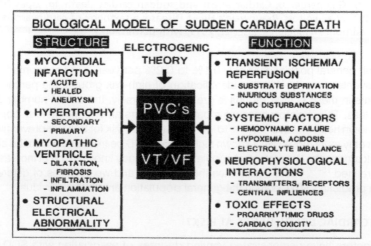

Fig. 1. Structure, function, and the pathogenesis of SCD. Biological model of SCD showing structure (substrate), function (trigger), and electrogenesis of VT or VF. PVC, premature ventricular contraction. (*Adapted from* Myerburg RJ, Kessler KM, Bassett AL, et al. A biological approach to sudden cardiac death: structure, function and cause. Am J Cardiol 1989;63(20):1513; with permission.)

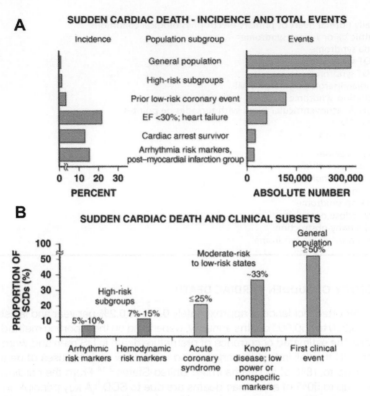

Fig. 2. Impact of population subgroups and time from events on the clinical epidemiology of SCD. (*A*) Estimates of incidence (%/year) and the total number of events per year for the general adult population in the United States and for increasingly high-risk subgroups. (*B*) Distribution of the clinical status of victims at the time of SCD. EF, ejection fraction. (*From* Myerburg RJ, Goldberger JJ. Cardiac arrest and sudden cardiac death. In: Zipes DP, Libby P, Bonow RO, et al, editors. Braunwald's Heart Disease: a textbook of cardiovascular medicine, 11th edition. Philadelphia: Elsevier; 2019; with permission.)

in the adult general population is only 0.1% to 0.2% per year, it still accounts for up to 450,000 events annually. With the identification of high-risk groups, the percentage of SCD events in these smaller groups is greater; conversely, the overall number of SCD events is less. This is simply because most SCD occurs among the general population without known heart disease.[15] Thus, to identify people at risk for SCD for preventive therapies, not only must those with a known high risk for SCD be treated but also the ability to detect risk among the larger general population not already known to be at increased risk must be refined.[15–17] **Table 1** illustrates the strengths and weaknesses of different risk factors in predicting SCD, both in the general population and in the individual.

SUDDEN CARDIAC DEATH: WHO'S AT RISK?

Several factors have demonstrated varying degrees of association with SCD. Some are intrinsic and immutable, whereas others are related to modifiable cardiovascular risk factors. Though the optimal combination of risk factors to identify patients at increased risk for SCD with high sensitivity or specificity remains the yet unreached holy grail for clinicians and scientists, it is generally understood that the number of

Table 1
Power cascade for risk prediction in sudden cardiac death

Strategy	Examples	Measures	Power
Conventional risk factors	Framingham risk index	Prediction of evolution of disease	High for the population Low for the individual
Anatomic disease screening	Coronary calcium score and computed tomography angiography	Identification of abnormal coronary arteries	High for anatomic identification Low for individual event prediction
Clinical risk profiling	Ejection fraction, stress testing, imaging techniques	Extent of disease	High for small, high-risk subgroups Low for large, low-risk subgroups
Transient risk predictors	Inflammatory markers; thrombotic cascade	Prediction of unstable plaques; acute changes in vascular status	Uncertain feasibility
Personalized risk predictors	Familial or genetic profiles	Individual SCD expression	Uncertain clinical precision; in evolution

Adapted from Myerburg RJ, Goldberger JJ. Cardiac arrest and sudden cardiac death. In: Zipes DP, Libby P, Bonow RO, et al, editors. Braunwald's Heart Disease: a textbook of cardiovascular medicine, 11th edition. Philadelphia: Elsevier; 2019; with permission.

risk factors present in an individual correlates with their overall risk. A list of common risk factors (see later discussion) is included in **Box 2**.

Immutable Risk Factors

Age
Etiologic factors causing SCD vary depending on an individual's age (**Fig. 3**A). There is a general increase in SCD risk beginning around age 35 years (incidence ~1/1000 person-years), which correlates with the increased prevalence of CHD over time.[18] Despite this, the number of CHD-attributable deaths due to SCD specifically decreases over the same time span. Furthermore, lifetime SCD risk in an analysis of Framingham Heart Study participants decreased beyond 75 years of age, compared with those at ages 45 to 55 years, exhibiting an inverse relationship with an individual's burden of comorbidities and competing modes of death.[19]

Sex
Overall, SCD exhibits a male preponderance in epidemiologic studies[20] (see **Fig. 3**B). For example, in the Framingham study noted previously, the lifetime SCD risk at each decade assessed was higher for men compared with women.[19] SCD incidence is nearly 4-fold to 7-fold greater in men compared with women before age 65 years, likely due to an increased incidence of CHD in men and the favorable cardiovascular effects conferred to premenopausal women.[3] Afterward, the odds of SCD remain around 2:1 for men, with progressive reduction in this difference over time. CHD is the most common cause of SCD in women older than age 40 years, and all the traditional CHD risk factors are implicated.[21] Despite this, women are 66% less likely to have known coronary artery disease (CAD) before SCD and 49% less likely to have known severe left ventricular (LV) dysfunction before SCD.[22] These findings suggest women are likely

Box 2
Sudden cardiac death risk factors
Age
Sex
Race
Activity level
Obesity
Hypertension
Glucose intolerance or diabetes mellitus
Elevated serum cholesterol
Decreased vital capacity
Smoking
Personal or family history of SCA
History of CAD
History of MI
History of ventricular tachycardia
Decreased LVEF less than or equal to 40%
Congestive heart failure
Left ventricular hypertrophy
Intraventricular conduction delay
Genetic arrhythmic and structural heart diseases
Heart rate variability

less often categorized as high risk for SCD and more often found to present with SCD as a first cardiovascular event.

Race

Though historical data regarding the association between race and SCD have been conflicting and should be interpreted with caution, some studies suggest a higher risk of SCD in blacks compared with whites.[23] In contrast, there seems to be a lower risk of SCD in the Hispanic population.[23] **Fig. 3**B demonstrates these relationships over time and with respect to sex.

Family History or Genetic Factors

A family history of cardiac arrest in a first-degree relative increases an individual's risk of cardiac arrest by 50%.[24] Heredity is another important feature of certain conditions predisposing to SCD and can be considered in 4 main categories[3,25]:

- Genetically based primary arrhythmia disorders: these are uncommon inherited arrhythmic syndromes (eg, congenital long QT syndrome [LQTS], Brugada syndrome [BrS]).
- Inherited structural heart disease with increased SCD risk: patients with conditions such as hypertrophic cardiomyopathy and arrhythmogenic right ventricular dysplasia/cardiomyopathy (ARVD/C) make up this category and require risk stratification to determine which individuals may benefit from intervention.

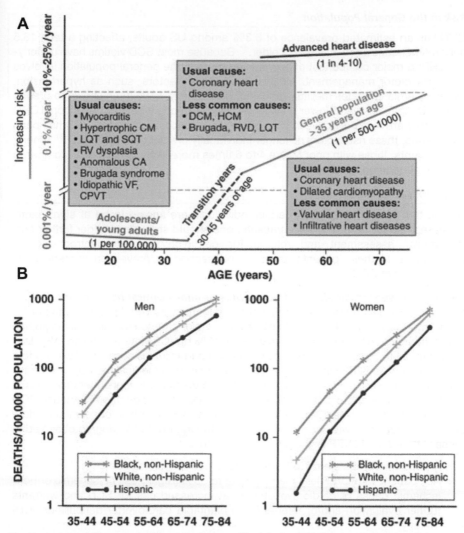

Fig. 3. Age-specific, sex-specific, and race-specific risks for SCD. (*A*) Age-related and disease-specific risk for SCD. (*B*) SCD risk as a function of age, sex, and race or culture (white, black, and Hispanic). CA, cardiac arrest; CM, cardiomyopathy; CPVT, catecholaminergic polymorphic VT; DCM, dilated CM; HCM, hypertrophic CM; LQT, long QT; RV, right ventricular; RVD, RV dysplasia; SQT, short QT. (*From* Myerburg RJ, Goldberger JJ. Cardiac arrest and sudden cardiac death. In: Zipes DP, Libby P, Bonow RO, et al, editors. Braunwald's Heart Disease: a textbook of cardiovascular medicine, 11th edition. Philadelphia: Elsevier; 2019; with permission.)

- Genetic predisposition to induced or secondary arrhythmias leading to SCD: these conditions include acquired LQTS, and electrolyte and metabolic derangements with genetic underpinnings.
- Genetic modulation of acquired diseases: diseases such as CAD and dilated cardiomyopathy due to genetic factors, which can occur in greater frequency in some families compared with the general population.

Risk in the General Population

CHD has an estimated prevalence of 6.3% among US adults, affecting a total 16.5 million Americans aged 20 years or older.[11] Because most SCD victims have underlying CHD, a major component of preventive efforts in the general population involves CHD risk factor management. Modifiable CHD risk factors, such as hypertension, hyperlipidemia, diabetes mellitus, smoking, and obesity, have been shown to predict SCD.[26] Despite an overall lower prevalence of CHD among women, conventional CHD risk factors are also predictive in this population.[20] Once overt clinical CHD has been established, these risk factors no longer individually predict the risk of SCD.[27] Among CHD patients, those with prior MI are 4 to 6 times more likely to have SCD compared with the general population.[28]

High Risk Factor Groups

Among the general population, certain individuals are known to be at significantly increased risk for SCD. For these patients, one should strongly consider further cardiovascular assessment and referral for cardiology and/or electrophysiology consultation. In these patients, primary and secondary prevention strategies are used to prevent SCD.

Reduced left ventricular ejection fraction plus or minus clinical heart failure

Reduced LV ejection fraction (LVEF) is the single most powerful predictive factor for overall mortality and SCD[3,29,30] and serves as a major criterion for determining appropriate therapy to prevent SCD. Approximately 45% of SCA victims have an LVEF less than or equal to 30%.[31] The presence of clinical heart failure is associated with up to a 5-fold increase in SCD risk.[28,32] Despite improvements in medical therapy, symptomatic heart failure still confers a 25% risk of SCD in the first 2.5 years after diagnosis.[33] SCD accounts for approximately 30% to 50% of heart failure deaths.[32] Although SCD risk is less studied in heart failure with preserved LVEF ($\geq$40%), observational data show an association with increased SCD risk, though not to the degree observed in those with reduced LVEF less than or equal to 40%.[34]

   Key populations for referral to Cardiologist/Electrophysiologist
   - Any patient with LVEF less than or equal to 35% (regardless of ischemic or nonischemic cause of cardiomyopathy) is at increased risk for SCD and warrants further evaluation and/or referral for implantable cardioverter-defibrillator (ICD) therapy
   - Patients with LVEF of 36% to 40%, with prior MI and documented nonsustained VT (NSVT; $\geq$3 consecutive PVCs) by Holter monitoring, electrocardiogram (ECG) tracing during a stress test, or any other modality, are at increased risk for SCD and warrant further evaluation and/or referral for ICD therapy
   - Specific recommendations regarding patients with ischemic heart disease and reduced LVEF at risk for SCD generally also apply to those with nonischemic cardiomyopathies (**Fig. 4**).[1]

Known or suspected ventricular arrhythmias

SCA survivors have an increased risk of recurrent events within the following 12 months,[35] and their risk of recurrent SCA continues to increase over time.[36] Furthermore, patients with underlying structural heart disease are at increased risk for VT or VF. This risk is typically modulated by the type, severity, and duration of structural disease, and is further increased in those with depressed LVEF and heart failure.[1] Finally, ventricular arrhythmias are an important cause of cardiac syncope. In studies of patients with unexplained, possibly arrhythmogenic, syncope, a finding

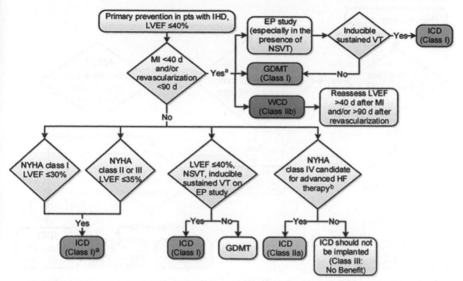

Fig. 4. Primary prevention of SCD in patients with ischemic heart disease. [a] Scenarios exist for early ICD placement in select circumstances, such as patients with a pacing indication or syncope. [b] Advanced HF therapy includes cardiac resynchronization therapy, cardiac transplant, and left ventricular assist device thought due to VT. EP, electrophysiological; GDMT, guideline-directed management and therapy; HF, heart failure; IHD, ischemic heart disease; NYHA, New York Heart Association; pts, patients; WCD, wearable cardioverter-defibrillator. (*Reprinted from* Heart Rhythm Volume 15, Issue 10, Al-Khatib SM, Stevenson WG, Ackerman, MJ, et al, 2017 AHA/ACC/HRS guideline for management of patients with ventricular arrhythmias and the prevention of sudden cardiac death: Executive summary A Report of the American College of Cardiology/American Heart Association Task Force on Clinical Practice Guidelines and the Heart Rhythm Society, e190–e252, Copyright 2018, with permission from Elsevier.)

of inducible VT at electrophysiology study was associated with a 48% rate of SCD at 3 years.[37]

Key populations for referral
- Any patient who has survived a SCA with no identified reversible cause (eg, severe hypokalemia or occurring within 48 hours of acute MI) should be referred for consideration of ICD implantation
- Patients with hemodynamically stable, sustained (≥30 seconds) monomorphic VT
- Patients with recurrent syncope concerning for an arrhythmogenic cause.

Hypertrophic cardiomyopathy
Hypertrophic cardiomyopathy (HCM) is "characterized by unexplained LV hypertrophy associated with non-dilated ventricular chambers in the absence of another cardiac or systemic disease that itself would be capable of producing the magnitude of hypertrophy evident in a given patient."[38] Among the approximately 1 in 500 individuals with unexplained LV hypertrophy, 20% to 30% have sarcomeric mutations consistent with clinically expressed HCM.[11,38] HCM is the most common cause of SCD in individuals younger than 40 years of age,[39] and 51% of HCM deaths are due to SCD.[40] Several SCD risk factors have been established for HCM patients (**Fig. 5**).

Key patients for referral with HCM[38]
- Survival from a cardiac arrest due to VT or VF
- Spontaneous sustained monomorphic VT causing syncope or hemodynamic compromise

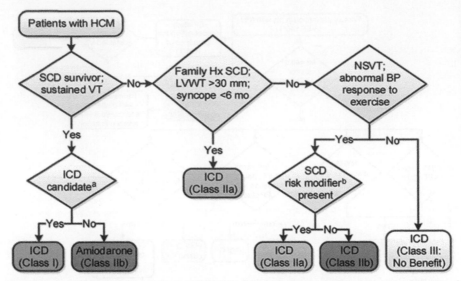

Fig. 5. Prevention of SCD in patients with HCM. [a] ICD candidacy as determined by functional status, life expectancy, or patient preference. [b] Risk modifiers: age less than 30 years, late gadolinium enhancement on cardiac MRI, LV outflow tract obstruction, LV aneurysm, syncope greater than 5 years. BP, blood pressure; Hx, history; LVWT, LV wall thickness. (*Reprinted from* Heart Rhythm Volume 15, Issue 10, Al-Khatib SM, Stevenson WG, Ackerman, MJ, et al, 2017 AHA/ACC/HRS guideline for management of patients with ventricular arrhythmias and the prevention of sudden cardiac death: Executive summary A Report of the American College of Cardiology/American Heart Association Task Force on Clinical Practice Guidelines and the Heart Rhythm Society, e190–e252, Copyright 2018, with permission from Elsevier.)

- Family history of SCD associated with HCM
- Maximal LV wall thickness greater than or equal to 30 mm by echocardiogram
- Unexplained syncope within the preceding 6 months
- Patients with NSVT or abnormal exercise response who also have 1 or more risk modifiers: age less than 30 years, delayed hyperenhancement on cardiac MRI, LV outflow tract obstruction, syncope greater than 5 years ago, and LV aneurysm.

Long QT syndrome

Congenital LQTS is a genetic channelopathy with an estimated prevalence of approximately 1 per 2000 births.[41] It is characterized by a prolonged QT interval, which renders individuals susceptible to syncope and SCD. Mutations in 15 genes have been linked to the LQTS phenotype.[42] Among these, long QT (LQT)-1 (KCNQ1, triggered by emotional or physical stress and activities such as swimming or diving), LQT2 (KCNH2, triggered by emotional stress, sudden arousal, auditory stimuli), and LQT3 (SCN5A, triggered at rest or during sleep) account for approximately 80% of known mutations.[43] Symptoms include palpitations and near-syncope or syncope, and the degree of QT prolongation increases the risk for adverse events.[41] The mainstay of medical therapy involves beta-adrenergic receptor blockade, which can decrease the SCD risk to 1% over 5 years in LQT1 patients, with reduced efficacy in LQT2 or LQT3.[44]

Key patients for referral with LQT
- Patients with a history of SCA
- Patients with recurrent syncope despite beta-blocker therapy
- Patients with severe QT prolongation without a secondary cause.[1]

Congenital LQTS is to be differentiated from acquired LQTS, which generally is a secondary phenomenon due to a drug side effect, electrolyte derangements, and/or bradycardia. Commonly implicated are antiarrhythmic, antipsychotic, and antibiotic drugs. Both congenital and acquired LQTS requires discontinuation of QT-prolonging medications, which are detailed at Web sites such as www. crediblemeds.org.

Brugada syndrome

BrS is an autosomal dominant channelopathy most often involving a loss-of-function SCN5A sodium channel mutation (15%–30% of cases), though numerous other sodium channel mutations, as well as mutations affecting calcium and potassium handling at the cellular level, have been identified.[45] BrS prevalence is estimated between 1 in 5000 and 1 in 2000, with an 8-fold to 10-fold higher prevalence in men compared with women.[46] Overall, BrS is thought to be responsible for up to 20% of SCD in structurally normal hearts. It has characteristic ECG findings of persistent ST-segment elevation in the precordial leads (V1-V3) and right bundle branch block, which are now classified into type 1 and type 2 patterns, with type 1 being the true diagnostic pattern and type 2 warranting further evaluation (**Fig. 6**). Importantly, aside from recognizing the characteristic ECG findings, there are many confounders of BrS due to conditions with similar ECG manifestations (eg, acute pulmonary embolism, ARVD/C), as well as modulating factors that may unmask a diagnostic BrS pattern, sometimes referred to as acquired BrS.[45,46] These modulators include medications that alter ionic currents at the cellular level (eg, lithium, tricyclic antidepressants), as well as febrile states.[46] In many cases, the unmasking may reflect an underlying channelopathy, which merits cardiology and/or electrophysiology referral for further investigation.[47] BrS therapy generally involves avoidance of fever and exacerbating medications. ICD therapy for SCD prevention is recommended in all patients with

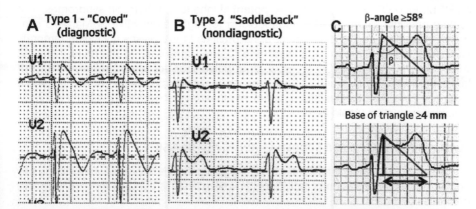

Fig. 6. Electrocardiographic patterns in BrS. (*A*) Type 1 Brugada ECG pattern showing a concave ST-segment elevation greater than or equal to 2 mm in greater than or equal to 1 right precordial lead, followed by a negative T-wave. (*B*) Type 2 Brugada ECG pattern showing a convex ST-segment elevation greater than or equal to 0.5 mm (generally ≥2 mm) in greater than or equal to 1 right precordial lead followed by a positive T-wave. (*C*) Additional criteria for the diagnosis of Brugada ECG pattern type 2 (*top*: the β angle, described by Chevallier and colleagues[59]; *bottom*: the length of the base triangle of the r′ wave 5 mm below the maximum rise point). (*From* Brugada J, Campuzano O, Arbelo E, et al. Present status of Brugada Syndrome: JACC state-of-the-art review. J Am Coll Cardiol 2018;72(9):1049; with permission.)

spontaneous type 1 ECG and a history of SCA, sustained ventricular arrhythmias or arrhythmic syncope.[1] Asymptomatic patients with only induced type 1 ECG patterns merit observation without therapy.

The preceding conditions are not exhaustive; however, they represent the high-risk groups most likely to be seen outside of specialized centers. Other patients at elevated risk for SCD are included in **Box 1**.

Sudden cardiac death risk in athletes

Sports-related SCD is defined as "sudden and unexpected death occurring during, or shortly after, exercise (with varying time intervals up to 24h used by different investigators), if witnessed by a bystander and/or happening in an individual who was otherwise known to be healthy."[48] It is estimated that 1 to 2 per 100,000 athletes between the ages of 12 and 35 years experience SCD annually.[48] In athletes younger than 35 years, HCM is the most common cause of SCD. However, for athletes older than 35 years, CHD is the most common cause.[3] In the US National Registry of Sudden Death in Athletes from 1980 to 2011, there were 1306 SCDs in young athletes (mean 19 ± 6 years of age) participating in organized sports. The most common causes of SCD in 842 young athletes with confirmed diagnoses were HCM (36%), coronary artery anomalies (19%), myocarditis (7%), arrhythmogenic right ventricular cardiomyopathy (5%), CAD (4%), and commotio cordis (3%).[49] Understanding the epidemiology of SCD in athletes lends itself to focusing on potential abnormalities that may be detected during routine evaluation. The routine evaluation would include a obtaining a medical history, physical exam and potentially an ECG. The medical history would include any symptoms such as exertional chest pain, exertional dyspnea, unexplained lightheadedness or syncope, or a prior history of any cardiac abnormalities, including hypertension, cardiac murmurs, etc. It would also include obtaining a detailed family history such as a history of premature sudden cardiac death in someone less than 50 years old or a family history of certain known cardiac conditions such as HCM, long QT, Marfan's, or other potential inherited arrhythmia syndromes. The routine physical exam would include looking for signs suggestive of Marfan's syndrome, including pectus excavatum, abnormalities in the pulses (including femoral), variations in blood pressure between the 2 arms and cardiac murmurs including with Valsalva maneuver. ON an ECG, one would look for preexcitation, LVH, prolonged QT interval, Brugada Pattern, epsilon wave, or conduction abnormalities. If even one portion of the described routine evaluation is abnormal then further cardiovascular evaluation would be warranted.[50]

EVALUATING PATIENTS FOR SUDDEN CARDIAC DEATH RISK

A focused but detailed history and physical examination is necessary to elicit the key details for risk stratification of individuals in whom there is concern for ventricular arrhythmias or SCA or SCD.

Patient history
- Symptoms related to heart disease in general: chest pain, dyspnea at rest or with exertion, orthopnea, paroxysmal nocturnal dyspnea, lower extremity edema
- Findings related to arrhythmic history: palpitations; lightheadedness or dizziness; chest tightness, fullness, or pressure; dyspnea or shortness of breath; syncope; cardiac arrest
- Temporal factors: onset or timing of symptoms or episodes, correlation with exercise, emotional stress
- Known heart disease: CHD, valvular disease, congenital disease, others

- Cardiovascular risk factors: hypertension, hyperlipidemia, diabetes mellitus, obesity, smoking, sleep apnea
- Medications: antiarrhythmic drugs (AADs), chronotropic agents, QT-prolonging medications, drug–drug interactions, stimulants (eg, cocaine, methamphetamines), supplements (eg, hormonal, steroids, over-the-counter)
- Medical history: thyroid disease, renal disease, electrolyte disturbances, stroke or embolic phenomena, lung disease, epilepsy, alcohol consumption, illicit substance use, unexplained motor vehicle crash.

Family history
- SCD, SCA, or unexplained drowning in a first-degree relative
- Sudden infant death syndrome or repetitive spontaneous pregnancy losses
- Heart disease: premature ischemic heart disease, cardiomyopathy (HCM, dilated, ARVD/C), congenital heart disease, cardiac channelopathies (BrS, LQTS, short QT, catecholaminergic polymorphic VT, arrhythmias, conduction disorders, required pacemaker or ICD)
- Neuromuscular diseases associated with cardiomyopathy or SCD: muscular dystrophy
- Epilepsy.

Physical examination
- Heart regularity and rate
- Blood pressure, jugular venous pressure
- Detectable murmurs
- Pulses and bruits
- Edema
- Sternotomy or other scars.

TREATMENT OF PATIENTS AT RISK FOR SUDDEN CARDIAC DEATH

Depending on an individual's risk profile, the treatment approach will vary with respect to preventing SCD. The following section outlines some general considerations for therapy.

General Population

In the general population, individuals may have identified SCD risk factors, which may be immutable or modifiable. The general goal in this population is to mitigate and control risk factors to prevent cardiovascular events, including SCD:

- Blood pressure control
- Optimal diabetes management
- Cholesterol management
- Smoking cessation
- Maintenance of a healthy body weight
- Exercise
- Stress management.

Existing Cardiovascular Disease

Individuals without manifest cardiovascular disease have additional goals for SCD prevention, beyond risk factor modification:

- Correction of ischemia: coronary revascularization; beta-adrenergic blockade (BB)
- Prevention of plaque rupture: aspirin; statin therapy; angiotensin-converting enzyme inhibitor (ACEi)

Table 2
Major implantable cardioverter-defibrillator trials for prevention of sudden cardiac death

Trial	Year	Subjects (n)	Inclusion Criterion: LVEF	Mode of Prevention	Hazard Ratio (95% CI)	P-Value
MADIT I	1996	196	≤35%	Primary	0.46 (0.26–0.82)	.009
AVID	1997	1016	≤40%	Secondary	0.62 (0.43–0.82)	<.02
MADIT II	2002	1232	≤30%	Primary	0.69 (0.51–0.93)	.016
DEFINITE	2004	485	<36%	Primary	0.65 (0.40–1.06)	.08
SCD-HeFT	2006	1676	≤35%	Primary	0.77 (0.62–0.96)	.007

Abbreviations: AVID, antiarrhythmics versus implantable defibrillators (AVID) trial; DEFINITE, defibrillators in non-ischemic cardiomyopathy treatment evaluation trial; MADIT I, multicenter automatic defibrillator implantation trial I; MADIT II, multicenter automatic defibrillator implantation trial II; SCD-HeFT, sudden cardiac death in heart failure trial.

- Stabilization of autonomic balance and neurohormonal blockade: BB; ACEi; aldosterone receptor blockade
- Improving LVEF: BB; ACEi
- Prevention of arrhythmias: BB; amiodarone.

Implantable Cardioverter-Defibrillator Therapies

Due to the association of frequent ventricular ectopy with SCD, multiple trials were carried out in the 1980s and 1990s to test the hypothesis that AAD therapy could effectively treat ventricular arrhythmias post-MI and prevent SCD; however, the data collectively do not support AAD use for prevention of SCD and, in some studies, they have been associated with increased harm.[51] On the other hand, ICD therapy, following initial trials for primary and secondary prevention,[35,52] has rapidly evolved into a highly efficacious therapy for the prevention of SCD in patients with a variety of indications. Notably, the benefits of ICD therapy are conferred even to patients already on maximally tolerated guideline-directed medical therapy (**Table 2**). A patient thought to be high risk who is referred to a cardiologist and/or electrophysiologist for further evaluation is likely to be considered for ICD implantation if she or he is an appropriate candidate.[1,29,53] Despite popular misconceptions, an ICD does not prevent SCA but rather treats it to prevent SCD. Furthermore, defibrillators have been shown to be more cost-effective per life years saved than coronary artery bypass graft surgery, medical therapy for hypertension, cardiac transplant, and peritoneal dialysis.[1,54–56]

For individuals whose treatment with a long-term implantable defibrillator is delayed, but are at increased risk of SCD, then an external wearable cardioverter-defibrillator may be reasonable short-term solution.[57] Finally, in patients who are candidates for ICD therapy but do not require pacing therapies for bradycardia or ventricular arrhythmia termination, the subcutaneous ICD is a safe and effective extravascular preventative treatment of SCD.[58]

SUMMARY

In the general population, effective SCD prevention consists of aggressive management of CHD risk factors. However, several higher risk groups have been clearly shown to benefit from treatments to reduce the incidence of sudden death. The largest of those high-risk groups includes individuals with LVEF less than or equal to 35%, regardless of ischemic or nonischemic cardiomyopathy. These patients should be referred for further cardiology and/or electrophysiology consultation and consideration of ICD implantation. To ensure success, it is of paramount importance to clearly explain the concepts of SCD risk and prevention such that patients fully comprehend the purpose of referral to a heart rhythm specialist.

REFERENCES

1. Al-Khatib SM, Stevenson WG, Ackerman MJ, et al. 2017 AHA/ACC/HRS guideline for management of patients with ventricular arrhythmias and the prevention of sudden cardiac death. Circulation 2018;138:e272–391.

2. Stecker EC, Reinier K, Marijon E, et al. Public health burden of sudden cardiac death in the United States. Circ Arrhythm Electrophysiol 2014;7:212–7.

3. Myerburg R, Goldberger J. Cardiac arrest and sudden cardiac death. In: Mann DL, Zipes DP, Libby P, et al, editors. Braunwald's heart disease: a Textbook of cardiovascular medicine. 11th edition. Philadelphia: Elsevier; 2019. p. 807–47.

4. Junttila MJ, Hookana E, Kaikkonen KS, et al. Temporal trends in the clinical and pathological characteristics of victims of sudden cardiac death in the absence of previously identified heart disease. Circ Arrhythm Electrophysiol 2016;9 [pii: e003723].

5. Fishman GI, Chugh SS, Dimarco JP, et al. Sudden cardiac death prediction and prevention: report from a National Heart, Lung, and Blood Institute and Heart Rhythm Society Workshop. Circulation 2010;122:2335–48.

6. Ni H, Coady S, Rosamond W, et al. Trends from 1987 to 2004 in sudden death due to coronary heart disease: the Atherosclerosis Risk in Communities (ARIC) study. Am Heart J 2009;157:46–52.

7. Fox CS, Evans JC, Larson MG, et al. Temporal trends in coronary heart disease mortality and sudden cardiac death from 1950 to 1999: the Framingham Heart Study. Circulation 2004;110:522–7.

8. Goldberger JJ, Buxton AE, Cain M, et al. Risk stratification for arrhythmic sudden cardiac death: identifying the roadblocks. Circulation 2011;123:2423–30.

9. Zheng ZJ, Croft JB, Giles WH, et al. Sudden cardiac death in the United States, 1989 to 1998. Circulation 2001;104:2158–63.

10. Buxton AE, Calkins H, Callans DJ, et al. ACC/AHA/HRS 2006 key data elements and definitions for electrophysiological studies and procedures: a report of the American College of Cardiology/American Heart Association task force on clinical data standards (ACC/AHA/HRS writing committee to develop data standards on electrophysiology). J Am Coll Cardiol 2006;48:2360–96.

11. Benjamin EJ, Virani SS, Callaway CW, et al. Heart disease and stroke statistics-2018 update: a report from the American Heart Association. Circulation 2018; 137:e67–492.

12. Hohnloser S, Weiss M, Zeiher A, et al. Sudden cardiac death recorded during ambulatory electrocardiographic monitoring. Clin Cardiol 1984;7:517–23.

13. Myerburg RJ, Kessler KM, Bassett AL, et al. A biological approach to sudden cardiac death: structure, function and cause. Am J Cardiol 1989;63:1512–6.

14. Kong MH, Fonarow GC, Peterson ED, et al. Systematic review of the incidence of sudden cardiac death in the United States. J Am Coll Cardiol 2011;57:794–801.

15. Myerburg RJ, Goldberger JJ. Sudden cardiac arrest risk assessment: population science and the individual risk mandate. JAMA Cardiol 2017;2:689–94.

16. Myerburg RJ, Kessler KM, Castellanos A. Sudden cardiac death. Structure, function, and time-dependence of risk. Circulation 1992;85:I2–10.

17. Wellens HJ, Schwartz PJ, Lindemans FW, et al. Risk stratification for sudden cardiac death: current status and challenges for the future. Eur Heart J 2014;35: 1642–51.
18. Myerburg RJ. Sudden cardiac death: exploring the limits of our knowledge. J Cardiovasc Electrophysiol 2001;12:369–81.
19. Bogle BM, Ning H, Mehrotra S, et al. Lifetime risk for sudden cardiac death in the community. J Am Heart Assoc 2016;5 [pii:e002398].
20. Kannel WB, Wilson PW, D'Agostino RB, et al. Sudden coronary death in women. Am Heart J 1998;136:205–12.
21. Albert CM, Chae CU, Grodstein F, et al. Prospective study of sudden cardiac death among women in the United States. Circulation 2003;107:2096–101.
22. Chugh SS, Uy-Evanado A, Teodorescu C, et al. Women have a lower prevalence of structural heart disease as a precursor to sudden cardiac arrest: the Ore-SUDS (Oregon Sudden Unexpected Death Study). J Am Coll Cardiol 2009;54: 2006–11.
23. Gillum RF. Sudden cardiac death in Hispanic Americans and African Americans. Am J Public Health 1997;87:1461–6.
24. Maron BJ, Doerer JJ, Haas TS, et al. Sudden deaths in young competitive athletes: analysis of 1866 deaths in the United States, 1980-2006. Circulation 2009;119:1085–92.
25. Friedlander Y, Siscovick DS, Weinmann S, et al. Family history as a risk factor for primary cardiac arrest. Circulation 1998;97:155–60.
26. Albert CM, Ruskin JN. Risk stratifiers for sudden cardiac death (SCD) in the community: primary prevention of SCD. Cardiovasc Res 2001;50:186–96.
27. Kannel WB, Cupples LA, D'Agostino RB. Sudden death risk in overt coronary heart disease: the Framingham Study. Am Heart J 1987;113:799–804.
28. Adabag AS, Therneau TM, Gersh BJ, et al. Sudden death after myocardial infarction. JAMA 2008;300:2022–9.
29. Priori SG, Blomstrom-Lundqvist C, Mazzanti A, et al. 2015 ESC guidelines for the management of patients with ventricular arrhythmias and the prevention of sudden cardiac death: the task force for the management of patients with ventricular arrhythmias and the prevention of sudden cardiac death of the European Society of Cardiology (ESC)Endorsed by: Association for European Paediatric and Congenital Cardiology (AEPC). Europace 2015;17:1601–87.
30. Goldberger JJ, Cain ME, Hohnloser SH, et al. American Heart Association/American College of Cardiology Foundation/Heart Rhythm Society Scientific Statement on Noninvasive Risk Stratification Techniques for Identifying Patients at Risk for Sudden Cardiac Death. A scientific statement from the American Heart Association Council on Clinical Cardiology Committee on Electrocardiography and Arrhythmias and Council on Epidemiology and Prevention. J Am Coll Cardiol 2008;52:1179–99.
31. de Vreede-Swagemakers JJ, Gorgels AP, Dubois-Arbouw WI, et al. Out-of-hospital cardiac arrest in the 1990's: a population-based study in the Maastricht area on incidence, characteristics and survival. J Am Coll Cardiol 1997;30:1500–5.
32. Kannel WB, Plehn JF, Cupples LA. Cardiac failure and sudden death in the Framingham Study. Am Heart J 1988;115:869–75.
33. Sweeney MO. Sudden death in heart failure associated with reduced left ventricular function: substrates, mechanisms, and evidence-based management, Part I. Pacing Clin Electrophysiol 2001;24:871–88.
34. Adabag S, Smith LG, Anand IS, et al. Sudden cardiac death in heart failure patients with preserved ejection fraction. J Card Fail 2012;18:749–54.

35. Antiarrhythmics versus Implantable Defibrillators (AVID) Investigators. A comparison of antiarrhythmic-drug therapy with implantable defibrillators in patients resuscitated from near-fatal ventricular arrhythmias. N Engl J Med 1997; 337:1576–84.
36. Nehme Z, Andrew E, Nair R, et al. Recurrent out-of-hospital cardiac arrest. Resuscitation 2017;121:158–65.
37. Bass EB, Elson JJ, Fogoros RN, et al. Long-term prognosis of patients undergoing electrophysiologic studies for syncope of unknown origin. Am J Cardiol 1988; 62:1186–91.
38. Gersh BJ, Maron BJ, Bonow RO, et al. 2011 ACCF/AHA guideline for the diagnosis and treatment of hypertrophic cardiomyopathy: executive summary: a report of the American College of Cardiology Foundation/American Heart Association Task Force on practice guidelines. Circulation 2011;124:2761–96.
39. Maron BJ, Shen WK, Link MS, et al. Efficacy of implantable cardioverter-defibrillators for the prevention of sudden death in patients with hypertrophic cardiomyopathy. N Engl J Med 2000;342:365–73.
40. Maron BJ, Olivotto I, Spirito P, et al. Epidemiology of hypertrophic cardiomyopathy-related death: revisited in a large non-referral-based patient population. Circulation 2000;102:858–64.
41. Priori SG, Wilde AA, Horie M, et al. HRS/EHRA/APHRS expert consensus statement on the diagnosis and management of patients with inherited primary arrhythmia syndromes: document endorsed by HRS, EHRA, and APHRS in May 2013 and by ACCF, AHA, PACES, and AEPC in June 2013. Heart Rhythm 2013;10:1932–63.
42. Bezzina CR, Lahrouchi N, Priori SG. Genetics of sudden cardiac death. Circ Res 2015;116:1919–36.
43. Wedekind H, Burde D, Zumhagen S, et al. QT interval prolongation and risk for cardiac events in genotyped LQTS-index children. Eur J Pediatr 2009;168: 1107–15.
44. Priori SG, Napolitano C, Schwartz PJ, et al. Association of long QT syndrome loci and cardiac events among patients treated with beta-blockers. JAMA 2004;292: 1341–4.
45. Skinner JR, Winbo A, Abrams D, et al. Channelopathies that lead to sudden cardiac death: clinical and genetic aspects. Heart Lung Circ 2019;28:22–30.
46. Brugada J, Campuzano O, Arbelo E, et al. Present status of Brugada syndrome: JACC state-of-the-art review. J Am Coll Cardiol 2018;72:1046–59.
47. Junttila MJ, Gonzalez M, Lizotte E, et al. Induced Brugada-type electrocardiogram, a sign for imminent malignant arrhythmias. Circulation 2008;117:1890–3.
48. Mont L, Pelliccia A, Sharma S, et al. Pre-participation cardiovascular evaluation for athletic participants to prevent sudden death: position paper from the EHRA and the EACPR, branches of the ESC. Endorsed by APHRS, HRS, and SOLAECE. Eur J Prev Cardiol 2017;24:41–69.
49. Maron BJ, Haas TS, Ahluwalia A, et al. Demographics and epidemiology of sudden deaths in young competitive athletes: from the United States National Registry. Am J Med 2016;129:1170–7.
50. Maron BJ, Thompson PD, Ackerman MJ, et al. Recommendations and considerations related to preparticipation screening for cardiovascular abnormalities in competitive athletes: 2007 update: a scientific statement from the American Heart Association Council on Nutrition, Physical Activity, and Metabolism: endorsed by the American College of Cardiology Foundation. Circulation 2007;115: 1643–2455.

51. Teo KK, Yusuf S, Furberg CD. Effects of prophylactic antiarrhythmic drug therapy in acute myocardial infarction. An overview of results from randomized controlled trials. JAMA 1993;270:1589–95.
52. Moss AJ, Hall WJ, Cannom DS, et al. Improved survival with an implanted defibrillator in patients with coronary disease at high risk for ventricular arrhythmia. Multicenter Automatic Defibrillator Implantation Trial Investigators. N Engl J Med 1996; 335:1933–40.
53. Epstein AE, DiMarco JP, Ellenbogen KA, et al. 2012 ACCF/AHA/HRS focused update incorporated into the ACCF/AHA/HRS 2008 guidelines for device-based therapy of cardiac rhythm abnormalities: a report of the American College of Cardiology Foundation/American Heart Association Task Force on Practice Guidelines and the Heart Rhythm Society. J Am Coll Cardiol 2013;61:e6–75.
54. Kupersmith J, Holmes-Rovner M, Hogan A, et al. Cost-effectiveness analysis in heart disease, Part III: Ischemia, congestive heart failure, and arrhythmias. Prog Cardiovasc Dis 1995;37:307–46.
55. Camm J, Klein H, Nisam S. The cost of implantable defibrillators: perceptions and reality. European Heart Journal 2007;28:392–7.
56. Stanton MS, Bell GK. Economic outcomes of implantable cardioverter-defibrillators. Circulation 2000;101:1067–74.
57. Piccini JP Sr, Allen LA, Kudenchuk PJ, et al. Wearable cardioverter-defibrillator therapy for the prevention of sudden cardiac death: a science advisory from the American Heart Association. Circulation 2016;133:1715–27.
58. Bardy GH, Smith WM, Hood MA, et al. An entirely subcutaneous implantable cardioverter-defibrillator. N Engl J Med 2010;363:36–44.
59. Chevallier S, Forclaz A, Tenkorang J, et al. New electrocardiographic criteria for discriminating between Brugada types 2 and 3 patterns and incomplete right bundle branch block. J Am Coll Cardiol 2011;58:2290–8.

Cardiac Implantable Electronic Device Therapy

Permanent Pacemakers, Implantable Cardioverter Defibrillators, and Cardiac Resynchronization Devices

Melanie M. Steffen, BSN, Jeffery S. Osborn, MD,
Michael J. Cutler, DO, PhD*

KEYWORDS

- Pacemaker • Implantable cardioverter defibrillator
- Cardiac resynchronization therapy

KEY POINTS

- Cardiac implantable electronic devices (CIEDs) provide lifesaving therapy for the treatment of bradyarrhythmias, ventricular tachyarrhythmias, and advanced systolic heart failure.
- Advances in CIED therapy have expanded the number of patients receiving permanent pacemakers, implantable cardioverter defibrillators, and cardiac resynchronization therapy devices.
- These devices improve quality of life and, in many cases, reduce mortality. However, limitations remain in the management of patients requiring CIED therapy.

INTRODUCTION

Since the first implantable cardiac pacemaker was patented in 1959 by Greatbatch and implanted in 1960,[1] there have been rapid advancements in the technology and in the effectiveness of cardiac implantable electronic devices (CIEDs). Currently, there are 3 primary classes of CIEDs:

1. Permanent pacemakers (PPM)
2. Implantable cardioverter defibrillators (ICD)
3. Cardiac resynchronization therapy (CRT) devices (PPM or ICD).

Disclosures: M.M. Steffen has none. J.S. Osborn is a consultant or speaker for Abbott Medical and Phillips and Spectranetics. M.J. Cutler is a consultant or on the advisory board for Johnson & Johnson and Biosense Webster.

Intermountain Heart Rhythm Specialist, Intermountain Medical Center, 5169 Cottonwood Street, Suite 510, Murray, UT 84107, USA
* Corresponding author. Intermountain Heart Rhythm Specialists, Intermountain Medical Center, Eccles Outpatient Care Center, 5169 Cottonwood Street, Suite 510, Murray, UT 84107.
E-mail address: michael.cutler@imail.org

Med Clin N Am 103 (2019) 931–943
https://doi.org/10.1016/j.mcna.2019.04.005
0025-7125/19/© 2019 Elsevier Inc. All rights reserved.

Pacemakers were originally developed to provide lifesaving fixed rate pacing during bradycardia. Since the inception of the original implantable PPM, significant technological advances have produced PPMs that can simulate the heart's normal automaticity and atrioventricular (AV) activation patterns. Additionally, modern PPMs have longer battery longevity and are able to increase pacing rate in response to physical activity.

In 1980, Michel Mirowski and colleagues[2] implanted the first ICD into a patient who had survived sudden cardiac arrest for the secondary prevention of subsequent cardiac arrest. At the time, this was a somewhat controversial treatment but has since become a leading therapy for the primary and secondary prevention of sudden cardiac arrest.[3]

During the 1990s, both basic and clinical research identified the ability of CRT (simultaneous pacing from the right and left ventricle; ie, biventricular pacing) to produce favorable myocardial remodeling, and to reduce morbidity and mortality in select heart failure patients. CIEDs are more common today owing to the expanded indications for implant and the growing evidence of efficacy.[3] Technological advances in CIEDs continue currently and have resulted in smaller devices with longer battery longevity and improved diagnostic capabilities.

PACEMAKERS
Indications

A PPM is implanted for symptomatic bradyarrhythmias. The primary indications for implantation of PPMs are mainly based on strong expert consensus because these indications were mostly developed before the era of the randomized controlled trial (RCT). In general, the most common indications for implantation of a PPM are for the management of sinus node dysfunction and second and third degree AV block. **Fig. 1** provides a summary of the 2018 guidelines from the American College of

	Sinus Node Dysfunction	AV Block	Other
Class I Implant is indicated	• Symptomatic SND • Symptomatic bradycardia as a result of required drug therapy	• Symptomatic 3rd or 2nd degree block • Symptomatic 3rd or 2nd degree bock as a result of required drug therapy • Asymptomatic 3rd degree, Mobitz type II or high-grade AV block • Neuromuscular disorders with 2nd or 3rd degree AV block (symptomatic or asymptomatic)	• Alternating bundle branch block • Syncope with bundle branch block and evidence of infra nodal bock during electrophysiology study
Class IIa Implant is reasonable	• Tachy-brady syndrome with symptomatic bradycardia • Symptomatic chronotropic incompetence	• Symptomatic 1st degree block • Symptomatic 2nd degree Mobitz type I	• Kearns-Sayre syndrome and conduction disorders • Epilepsy with severe symptomatic bradycardia not effectively managed with medication
Class IIb Implant may be considered	• A trial of theophylline may be considered in likely symptomatic bradycardia to help evaluate the benefit of permanent pacing	• Neuromuscular disease with PR interval >240 ms, QRS duration >120 ms, or fascicular block	• Anderson-Fabry disease and QRS >110 ms
Class III Implant not indicated	• Asymptomatic SND • Symptoms do not correlate with SND and are present in the absence of bradycardia • Sleep related bradycardia or transient sinus pauses during sleep with no other indications for pacing	• Asymptomatic 1st degree block • Asymptomatic 2nd degree type I block • If the block is expected to resolve and not recur	• Bifascicular block without AV block or symptoms • Asymptomatic fascicular block with first degree AV block • Hypersensitive cardioinhibitory response to carotid sinus stimulation with no or minimal symptoms • Situational vasovagal syncope that can be managed with avoidance behavior

Fig. 1. Indications for permanent cardiac pacing. SND, sinus node dysfunction. (*Adapted from* Kusumoto FM, Schoenfeld MH, Barrett C, et al. 2018 ACC/AHA/HRS guideline on the evaluation and management of patients with bradycardia and cardiac conduction delay: a report of the American College of Cardiology/American Heart Association Task Force on Clinical Practice Guidelines and the Heart Rhythm Society. Heart Rhythm 2018; with permission.)

Cardiology, American Heart Association, and the Heart Rhythm Society (ACC/AHA/HRS) for the utilization of PPMs in the treatment of bradycardia.[4]

Pacemaker Leads and Generators

A pacemaker consists of the pulse generator (**Fig. 2**A) and the pacing leads (see **Fig. 2**B), which are connected to the pulse generator. Pacemaker leads consist of a small electrode at the distal end of the lead that is used for pacing and sensing. They have a fixation device (active or passive) at the distal tip for anchoring the lead to the myocardium. The proximal end of the lead connects to the pacemaker generator. The PPM generator consists of a titanium can that houses the electronic circuitry and battery that is attached to a plastic header where the proximal lead terminals attach to the generator.

The generator generally is placed between the subcutaneous tissue and pectoral fascia of the left upper chest. The leads are inserted transvenous through the

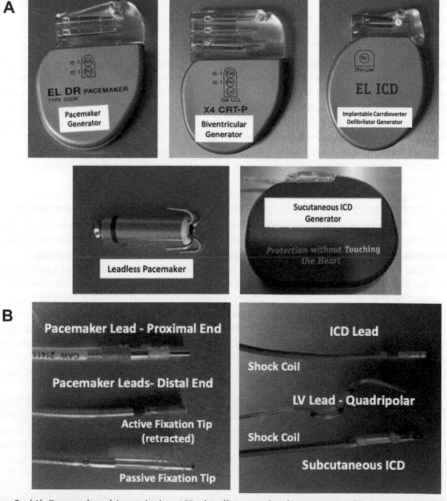

Fig. 2. (A) Pacemaker, biventricular, ICD, leadless, and subcutaneous ICD generators. (B) Pacemaker and ICD leads.

subclavian, axillary, or cephalic veins, and guided via fluoroscopy through the superior vena cava. An atrial lead is secured in the right atrial appendage. A ventricular lead is most commonly secured in the right ventricular (RV) apex. Good placement of pacemaker leads allows for low stimulation thresholds and adequate sensing of intrinsic electrical signals.

Leadless Pacemaker

The latest development in pacemaker technology is the single-chamber leadless PPM (see **Fig. 2**A). In this PPM there is no traditional pulse generator and no transvenous leads. The entire PPM is housed in a capsule that sits in the RV apex. It is implanted with a catheter through the femoral vein and deployed in the right ventricle. Advantages are that there is no PPM pocket that could become infected and that the lead component, which can fracture or develop insulation breaks, is eliminated. A disadvantage is that this technology is currently only available to pace the ventricle and, therefore, is most appropriate for patients with permanent atrial fibrillation. Also, because this is new technology, it is still unclear how many of these can be implanted in an individual's lifetime and how difficult they will be to extract if needed.

Basic Pacemaker Function and Programming

All pacemakers have 2 basic functions: (1) to pace and (2) to sense intrinsic electrical activity of the heart. In the United States, the most common type of implanted PPM is a dual-chamber device,[5] in which a lead is secured in the right atrium and a second lead in the right ventricle. A dual-chamber device is necessary with complete heart block or other types of AV block to allow for AV synchrony. The ventricular lead will pace in response to the sensed atrial activity, up to the programmed upper tracking rate. An atrial lead is required in sick sinus syndrome and chronotropic incompetence. Also, a ventricular lead is often placed in these patients in case they develop AV conduction disease in the future.[6]

A single-chamber pacemaker is generally placed in patients with symptomatic bradycardia secondary to AV block in the setting of chronic or permanent atrial fibrillation. In these cases, a single lead will be placed in the right ventricle. Less commonly, a single lead can be placed in the right atrium in the setting of sinus node dysfunction or chronotropic incompetence if there is no evidence of AV conduction delay.

Pacemakers are programmed based on the indication for implant and customized to the individual needs of each patient. They can be reprogrammed as needed. A lower rate limit is programmed at which the pacemaker will initiate a pacing impulse if no intrinsic rhythm is sensed above this rate. An upper rate is set that restricts the highest rate that the pacemaker will track the native atrial rate with beat-to-beat ventricular pacing in the setting of AV block. Higher heart rates than the maximum pacing rate can be seen if the native atrial (with intact AV conduction) or ventricular rate is faster than the programmed rate. The pacemaker will not prevent faster intrinsic heart rates.

Most pacemakers are programmed to inhibit pacing when they sense native electrical activity and only pace in the absence of intrinsic electrical activity. More specifically, pacemakers can be programmed to set which chamber or chambers will pace, which chamber or chambers will sense intrinsic electrical activity, how the pacemaker will respond to sensed electrical activity (ie, inhibit pacing), and if rate-adaptive pacing will be used. The North American Society of Pacing and Electrophysiology and British Pacing and Electrophysiology Group Generic (NBG) code is the international system used to describe pacemaker modes (**Table 1**).[7] The first column indicates what chamber or chambers are being paced. The second column represents the chamber or

Table 1
North American Society of Pacing and Electrophysiology and British Pacing and Electrophysiology Group generic code for pacing

I Chambers(s) Paced	II Chambers(s) Sensed	III Response to Sensing	IV Rate Modulation
O = None	O = None	O = None	O = None
A = Atrium	A = Atrium	T = Triggered	R = Rate modulation
V = Ventricle	V = Ventricle	I = Inhibit	
D = Dual (A+V)	D = Dual (A+V)	D = Dual (T+I)	

Adapted from Bernstein AD, Daubert JC, Fletcher RD, et al. The revised NASPE/BPEG generic code for antibradycardia, adaptive-rate, and multisite pacing. North American Society of Pacing and Electrophysiology/British Pacing and Electrophysiology Group. Pacing Clin Electrophysiol 2002;25(2):260–4; with permission.

chambers being sensed. The third column provides the pacemaker's response to sensed electrical activity. If the fourth column contains the letter R, it indicates rate-adaptive pacing is being used. Otherwise, if the fourth column is omitted, rate-adaptive pacing is not being used. Rate-adaptive pacing responds to sensors in the pacemaker to increase the heart rate during activity. The current rate-adaptive sensors are accelerometers that respond to movement and minute ventilation sensors that respond to increased respiratory rate.

IMPLANTABLE CARDIOVERTER DEFIBRILLATORS
Indications

In contrast to permanent pacing indications, the current guidelines for implantation of ICDs are based on robust data from multiple RCTs.[8–11] Initially, ICDs were primarily implanted for the secondary prevention of sudden cardiac arrest in patients who survived a cardiac arrest from a nonreversible cause. Subsequently, the results of landmark trials demonstrating the efficacy of ICD therapy for the primary prevention of sudden cardiac arrest in patients with ischemic and nonischemic cardiomyopathies have expanded the indications for ICD implantation. Overall, these studies have shown a 23% to 54% reduction in mortality in at-risk patients receiving an ICD versus medical therapy alone.[3] However, recent research has suggested that the benefit of ICD therapy in nonischemic cardiomyopathy patients is less clear than originally believed.[12] **Fig. 3** provides a summary of the current guidelines from ACC/AHA/HRS for the utilization of ICD therapy for the prevention of sudden cardiac arrest.[13]

Implantable Cardioverter Defibrillator Lead and Generators

Similar to a pacemaker, an ICD consists of the pulse generator and the pacing-ICD leads, which are connected to the pulse generator (see **Fig. 2**). In contrast to pacemaker leads, ICD leads also have 1 to 2 shocking coils incorporated into the body of the lead to allow for defibrillation. The ICD generator is generally larger than a pacemaker generator to accommodate the additional battery size and electrical circuitry needed for the defibrillation function of the device.

Subcutaneous Implantable Cardioverter Defibrillator

An alternative to the traditional transvenous ICD is the subcutaneous ICD (S-ICD). In this device, there are no transvenous leads implanted in the heart. The generator is implanted under the subcutaneous tissue on the left rib cage at the midaxillary line with a shock electrode that is tunneled in the subcutaneous tissue, along the sternum.

	Ventricular Arrhythmia	Heart Failure	Other
Class I Implant is indicated	• Survivor of cardiac arrest caused by VF or VT without reversible cause • Structural heart disease with spontaneous sustained VT • Unexplained syncope with hemodynamically significant VT or VF during electrophysiology study	• LVEF ≤35% in NYHA class II or III and have not had an MI within 40 days • LVEF ≤30% in NYHA class I and are more than 40 days post MI • NSVT due to prior MI with LVEF ≤40% and inducible VF or sustained VT in electrophysiology study	
Class IIa Implant is reasonable	• Sustained VT with normal ventricular function	• Unexplained syncope with significant LV dysfunction, and DCM	• HCM with at least 1 risk factor for SCD • ARVD with at least 1 risk factor for SCD • Long-QT syndrome with syncope or VT while on beta blockers • Awaiting heart transplant and not hospitalized • Brugada syndrome with syncope or documented VT • Catecholaminergic polymorphic VT with syncope or sustained VT while on beta blocker • Cardiac sarcoidosis, giant cell myocarditis, Chagas disease
Class IIb Implant may be considered		• LVEF ≤35% in NYHA class I • Familial cardiomyopathy associated with sudden death	• Long-QT syndrome with risk factors for SCD • Unexplained syncope with advanced structural heart disease • LV noncompaction
Class III Implant not indicated	• Incessant VT or VF • Unexplained syncope without inducible ventricular arrhythmias • VT or VF is receptive to ablation • VT or VF caused by reversible disorder	• NYHA class IV refractory to drug therapy and not a candidate for transplant or CRT-D	• Estimated survival is < 1 year regardless of if they meet implant criteria above • Significant psychiatric illness that would be aggravated by implant

Fig. 3. Indications for ICD. CRT-D, cardiac resynchronization therapy–ICD; LV, left ventricular; LVEF, LV ejection fraction; VT, ventricular tachycardia. (*Adapted from* Tracy CM, Epstein AE, Darbar D, et al. 2012 ACCF/AHA/HRS Focused Update of the 2008 Guidelines for Device-Based Therapy of Cardiac Rhythm Abnormalities: a report of the American College of Cardiology Foundation/American Heart Association Task Force on Practice Guidelines. Heart Rhythm 2012;9(10):1737–53; and Al-Khatib SM, Stevenson WG, Ackerman MJ, et al. 2017 AHA/ACC/HRS Guideline for Management of Patients With Ventricular Arrhythmias and the Prevention of Sudden Cardiac Death: Executive Summary: A Report of the American College of Cardiology/American Heart Association Task Force on Clinical Practice Guidelines and the Heart Rhythm Society. Circulation 2018; 138(13): e210–e271.)

This type of device is only for patients who do not have indications for pacing. It should be noted that S-ICDs cannot provide antitachycardia pacing (ATP). The advantage of the S-ICD is there are no intravenous (IV) leads. This eliminates some of the risks associated with IV implant, such as perforation, endocardial infection, or the potential need of a high-risk lead extraction in the future. It is particularly attractive in a younger patient population at risk of sudden death.

Basic Implantable Cardioverter Defibrillator Function and Programming

The main purpose of an ICD is to appropriately detect ventricular arrhythmias and deliver lifesaving therapy with ATP and/or defibrillation. Recent research has demonstrated that less aggressive ICD therapy programming reduces the incidence of inappropriate ICD shocks and reduces all-cause mortality when compared with more aggressive programming.[14]

ATP consists of pacing delivered at a shorter cycle length (ie, faster) than the ventricular arrhythmia itself. ATP has been shown to be highly effective in terminating both slow and fast ventricular tachycardia (VT).[15] Programmed shocks are aborted if the ATP is successful. ICDs can be programmed to have different therapies at different heart rates. A therapy zone can be set to only deliver ATP with no shocks or ATP with programmed shocks if ATP is not successful in terminating the ventricular arrhythmia. Using ATP does carry a small risk of accelerating the VT into a faster VT or ventricular fibrillation. This makes it essential to program shocks in a faster rate zone if a slower zone does not have shocks programmed. A monitor-only zone can also be programmed. In this zone, no therapies will be delivered regardless of the duration of the arrhythmia.

The most important job of an ICD is to appropriately treat ventricular arrhythmias. However, it is also important for the device to inhibit therapy when not needed, as in the case of atrial tachyarrhythmias such as atrial fibrillation with a rapid ventricular response. Recent research has identified an increased mortality associated with shocks, regardless of whether the shocks are appropriate or inappropriate.[16]

Atrial fibrillation with rapid ventricular response is a common cause of inappropriate ICD shocks. The rapid heart rate can be classified in the VT therapy zone and ATP is rarely effective in slowing the ventricular rate during atrial tachyarrhythmias. This then can lead to an inappropriate shock. To avoid shocks for atrial arrhythmias, discriminator functions of varying effectiveness can be programmed in the device.

CARDIAC RESYNCHRONIZATION THERAPY

Important research findings have identified the role of intraventricular conduction delay and its associated electrical dyssynchrony on the natural history of systolic heart failure.[17–19] These observations heralded in the development of CRT as a major treatment modality for the management of patients with systolic heart failure.[20] CRT, also known as biventricular pacing, generally consists of simultaneous pacing from the right and left ventricles and can be incorporated into either a PPM or an ICD. As the name implies, a pacing-ICD lead is placed in the right ventricle and an additional pacing lead is placed in the region of the left ventricle. The left ventricular (LV) lead is generally guided through the coronary sinus (CS) and through an accessible branch of the CS to attach to the lateral wall of the left ventricle.

The goal of CRT is to electrically resynchronize the left and right side of the heart to improve mechanical dyssynchrony that exists between the ventricular septum and the LV lateral wall. This is manifested on the electrocardiogram by the presence of a left bundle branch block. CRT has been associated with improved ejection fraction (EF), decreased heart failure events, improvement in the class of heart failure, and reduction in mortality.[21]

Indications

To be considered for CRT, heart failure patients with an LV EF less than or equal to 35% must be treated with guideline-directed medical therapy for 90 days without adequate improvement in EF and have a wide QRS (>120 ms). The guidelines to qualify for a biventricular device are strict and differ between a biventricular pacemaker and biventricular ICD. **Fig. 4** provides a summary of the current guidelines from ACC/AHA/HRS for the utilization of CRT.[22]

Left Ventricular Lead Placement

Placement of LV leads is often limited by the anatomy of the CS and the available coronary vein branches of the main CS. The development of quadripolar LV leads has helped mitigate these limitations. A quadripolar lead has 4 spaced electrodes along the distal end of the lead (see **Fig. 2B**). This aids in programming a pacing vector that optimizes the pacing threshold and QRS narrowing. When a patient does not have suitable CS anatomy, a pacing lead can be placed on the epicardial surface of the left ventricle using a minimally invasive surgical approach through a lateral thoracotomy.

	NHYA Class I	NYHA Class II	NYHA Class III and Ambulatory class IV	Other
Class I Implant is indicated		• LVEF ≤35% • QRS ≥150 ms • LBBB • Sinus rhythm	• LVEF ≤35% • QRS ≥150 ms • LBBB • Sinus rhythm	
Class IIa Implant is reasonable		• LVEF ≤35% • QRS 120-149 ms • LBBB • Sinus rhythm	• LVEF ≤35% • QRS 120-149 ms with LBBB or QRS ≥150 ms with no LBBB • Sinus rhythm	• Expected to require > 40% ventricular pacing • Atrial fibrillation and pacing is indicated with rate control resulting in near 100% pacing with CRT
Class IIb Implant may be considered	• LVEF ≤30% • QRS ≥150 ms • LBBB • Ischemic cardiomyopathy	• LVEF ≤35% • QRS ≥150 mg • No LBBB • Sinus Rhythm	• LVEF ≤35% • QRS 120-149 ms • No LBBB • Sinus Rhythm	
Class III Implant not indicated	• QRS ≤150 ms • No LBBB	• QRS ≤ 150 ms • No LBBB		

Fig. 4. Indications for CRT. To qualify for CRT, a patient must be on GDMT for greater than 90 days and be more than 40 days post-MI. (*Adapted from* Tracy CM, Epstein AE, Darbar D, et al. 2012 ACCF/AHA/HRS focused update of the 2008 guidelines for device-based therapy of cardiac rhythm abnormalities: a report of the American College of Cardiology Foundation/American Heart Association Task Force on Practice Guidelines. Heart Rhythm 2012;9(10):1737–53; with permission.)

Multipoint Pacing

About 25% of patients with CRT devices do not respond positively to therapy.[3] The recent development of multipoint pacing (MPP) has offered a new tool to use in non-responders to CRT. In MPP, the left ventricle is paced from 2 sites. By pacing from 2 sites, more myocardium is recruited to aid in resynchronization. The use of MPP has shown to produce a greater improvement in EF than traditional CRT.[23] This has been particularly beneficial for ischemic cardiomyopathy patients who have areas of scar that cannot propagate an electrical impulse.

His Bundle Pacing

RV apical pacing has been associated with worsening heart failure symptoms and the development of a pacing-mediated cardiomyopathy in patients who have an RV pace greater than 40% of the time. His bundle pacing provides an alternative to RV pacing that may mitigate the deleterious effect of RV pacing on LV function. Heart failure symptoms and admissions have been shown to be reduced.[24] This may be also be an alternative to biventricular pacing in patients with RV pacing–induced cardiomyopathy.[25]

COMPLICATIONS RELATED TO PACEMAKERS AND IMPLANTABLE CARDIOVERTER DEFIBRILLATORS
Infection

Postoperative infections are a significant complication and need immediate attention. Infections generally appear within 2 weeks of implant but can manifest greater than 6 months postprocedure. The risk of infection is higher during generator replacement procedure than with initial device implants.[6] This makes optimizing battery longevity, and thus decreasing the number of generator changes in a lifetime, essential in decreasing device-related infection. Superficial infections can be treated promptly with oral antibiotics. In contrast, deep pocket infections require that the generator and leads be explanted in conjunction with IV antibiotic therapy.[26] Prophylactic IV antibiotics given preprocedure have shown to decrease the occurrence of infection.[26,27] Although effective for the implant, prophylactic antibiotic use is not necessary before other medical or dental procedures after implant of a CIED.

Lead Failure

Pacemaker and ICD leads can fail over time secondary to insulation breaks and wire fractures. Thus, patients who have a CIED implanted at a young age will likely need 1 or more lead revision or replacement in their lifetimes. When leads fail it may be necessary to extract the leads. Abandoning leads can be undesirable secondary to possible venous occlusion and the increased complexity of future lead extraction. Advances in both mechanical and laser lead extraction tools have improved the success and safety of lead extraction. However, lead extraction still remains a high-risk procedure due to the possibility of life-threatening complications. In high-risk patients, such as the elderly, it is often advised to abandon the old lead and place a new lead when possible.

Hematoma

A pocket hematoma is a common postoperative complication. Generally, these are small enough that they will resolve without intervention. They do increase the risk of infection and, in some cases, antibiotic therapy is used to prevent pocket infections.[6] Rarely, a hematoma will be significant enough that the pocket must be reopened and the hematoma evacuated.

Cardiac Perforation

In rare cases, placement of a pacemaker-ICD lead can lead to cardiac perforation. This can, in turn, cause a pericardial effusion with or without pericardial tamponade. Microperforations generally do not have any clinical sequelae. Patients should be monitored for symptoms of pericardial effusion or tamponade. In the case of a slow leak, symptoms may not develop for 24 to 48 hours postprocedure.

Pacing-Induced Cardiomyopathy

Patients who require a high percentage of ventricular pacing (generally >40%) should be monitored for the development of cardiomyopathy. RV pacing can cause mechanical dyssynchrony, which can lead to systolic dysfunction. The treatment in these cases is to upgrade the device to a biventricular device. The exact incidence of this entity is unknown.

Phrenic Nerve Stimulation

A common complication of LV pacing and, less commonly, right atrial pacing is phrenic nerve or diaphragmatic stimulation. Although not harmful, it can be quite bothersome and intolerable for patients, depending on the severity. Patients often describe feeling a hiccup or a thumping sensation in their diaphragm. Often, the device can be reprogrammed to avoid stimulation of the phrenic nerve without repositioning the lead. However, in some cases the pacing lead must be repositioned to remedy the problem.

LONG-TERM DEVICE MANAGEMENT

It is generally recommended that pacemakers are checked every 6 to 12 months and ICDs are checked every 3 to 6 months.[28] This can be completed as an in-office check or with a remote monitor. A remote monitor uses radio frequency telemetry to communicate wirelessly with the CIED. Remote monitors can read battery longevity estimates, recorded arrhythmias, and lead data. This can result in earlier detection and treatment of device malfunction and arrhythmias, such as atrial fibrillation. It allows for device evaluation without the expense and time of an in-office visit. Currently, reprogramming is not possible using a remote monitor and an in-office visit is needed if device reprogramming is required.

COMMON CONCERNS RELATED TO CARDIAC IMPLANTABLE ELECTRONIC DEVICES

Pacemaker-Mediated Tachycardia

Pacemaker-mediated tachycardia (PMT) can be confused for VT. Some patients are symptomatic with PMT due to the inappropriate increase in heart rate and loss of AV synchrony. PMT most commonly occurs when there is retrograde electrical conduction from the ventricle to the atrium during a ventricular premature beat. The retrograde signal is sensed by the atrial lead as a normal electrical signal. The pacemaker will then deliver a pacing impulse to the ventricle in response to the sensed atrial signal. This cycle will continue at the maximum tracking rate. A quick temporary fix is to place a magnet over the pacemaker to put it in a nonsensing mode and pace in the atrium and ventricle at the programmed magnet rate. A permanent fix requires reprogramming a refractory period in the pacemaker so that the retrograde atrial signal is not sensed as a normal sinus signal.

End of Life Device Management

ICD management at the end of life is fairly straight forward and universally accepted. It is advisable to deactivate ICD therapies at the end of life to prevent painful shocks and allow the patient to pass peacefully. However, end of life management of pacemakers can create complex ethical dilemmas. The HRS has published an expert consensus document to assist in managing these situtations.[29]

Appropriate Imaging in Cardiac Implantable Electronic Device Patients

Radiographic, computed tomography, mammography, and ultrasound imaging can all be safely performed in patients with implanted cardiac devices. In the past, the presence of a CIED has been considered a contraindication for MRI. MRI conditional generators and leads have been developed and are available for implant. Case reviews and studies have shown it is safe to perform MRI in non-MRI conditional devices at facilities with appropriate guideline-directed protocols for management of these patients.[30]

Magnet Response

In ICDs, a magnet placed over the device will deactivate therapies while the magnet is in place without altering pacing function. When the magnet is removed, programmed therapies will resume. In contrast, a magnet placed over a pacemaker will result in the pacemaker switching to a nonsensing and continuous pacing mode at a fixed rate. As with an ICD, once the magnet is removed, the pacemaker will resume previous programming.

Electromagnetic Interference

The potential risk with electromagnetic interference (EMI) is inhibition of pacing or inappropriate ICD shocks. Bipolar sensing and improved filtering in modern CIEDs have greatly decreased the risk of EMI. There is little concern with EMI in general activities of daily living. Interference from microwaves is no longer a concern. Normal cell phone use is safe but it is recommended to keep the cell phone further than 8 cm from the device.[31] The greatest potential for EMI is within a medical environment.[31] Electrocautery is a large source of EMI and devices should be reprogrammed for medical procedures using electrocautery.

Pseudomalfunction

In-hospital telemetry tracings can show what appears to be abnormal pacemaker function due to unexplained pacing rates or timing. These can often be explained by programming algorithms and timings set in the pacemaker itself. It is important to have these investigated with a full device interrogation to differentiate true device malfunction from a pseudomalfunction.

SUMMARY

Advances in CIED therapy have expanded the number of patients receiving PPMs, ICDs, and CRT devices. These devices provide lifesaving therapies; have improved quality of life; and, in many cases, have reduced mortality. However, limitations remain in the management of patients who require CIED therapy. Technological advances in areas such as leadless devices, MPP, and improved battery longevity have begun to remedy many of the limitations of traditional devices.

REFERENCES

1. Beck H, Boden WE, Patibandla S, et al. 50th Anniversary of the first successful permanent pacemaker implantation in the United States: historical review and future directions. Am J Cardiol 2010;106:810–8.
2. Mirowski M, Reid PR, Mower MM, et al. Termination of malignant ventricular arrhythmias with an implanted automatic defibrillator in human beings. N Engl J Med 1980;303:322–4.
3. van Welsenes GH, Borleffs CJ, van Rees JB, et al. Improvements in 25 years of implantable cardioverter defibrillator therapy. Neth Heart J 2011;19:24–30.
4. Kusumoto FM, Schoenfeld MH, Barrett C, et al. 2018 ACC/AHA/HRS guideline on the evaluation and management of patients with bradycardia and cardiac conduction delay: a report of the American College of Cardiology/American Heart Association Task Force on Clinical Practice Guidelines and the Heart Rhythm Society. Heart Rhythm 2018. [Epub ahead of print].
5. Greenspon AJ, Patel JD, Lau E, et al. Trends in permanent pacemaker implantation in the United States from 1993 to 2009: increasing complexity of patients and procedures. J Am Coll Cardiol 2012;60:1540–5.
6. Polyzos KA, Konstantelias AA, Falagas ME. Risk factors for cardiac implantable electronic device infection: a systematic review and meta-analysis. Europace 2015;17:767–77.
7. Bernstein AD, Daubert JC, Fletcher RD, et al. The revised NASPE/BPEG generic code for antibradycardia, adaptive-rate, and multisite pacing. North American Society of Pacing and Electrophysiology/British Pacing and Electrophysiology Group. Pacing Clin Electrophysiol 2002;25:260–4.
8. Moss AJ, Hall WJ, Cannom DS, et al. Improved survival with an implanted defibrillator in patients with coronary disease at high risk for ventricular arrhythmia. Multicenter Automatic Defibrillator Implantation Trial Investigators. N Engl J Med 1996; 335:1933–40.

9. Moss AJ, Zareba W, Hall WJ, et al. Prophylactic implantation of a defibrillator in patients with myocardial infarction and reduced ejection fraction. N Engl J Med 2002;346:877–83.

10. Buxton AE, Lee KL, Fisher JD, et al. A randomized study of the prevention of sudden death in patients with coronary artery disease. Multicenter Unsustained Tachycardia Trial Investigators. N Engl J Med 1999;341:1882–90.

11. Bardy GH, Lee KL, Mark DB, et al. Amiodarone or an implantable cardioverter-defibrillator for congestive heart failure. N Engl J Med 2005;352:225–37.

12. Kober L, Thune JJ, Nielsen JC, et al. Defibrillator implantation in patients with nonischemic systolic heart failure. N Engl J Med 2016;375:1221–30.

13. Al-Khatib SM, Stevenson WG, Ackerman MJ, et al. 2017 AHA/ACC/HRS guideline for management of patients with ventricular arrhythmias and the prevention of sudden cardiac death: executive summary: a report of the American College of Cardiology/American Heart Association Task Force on Clinical Practice Guidelines and the Heart Rhythm Society. J Am Coll Cardiol 2018;72:1677–749.

14. Moss AJ, Schuger C, Beck CA, et al. Reduction in inappropriate therapy and mortality through ICD programming. N Engl J Med 2012;367:2275–83.

15. Wathen MS, DeGroot PJ, Sweeney MO, et al. Prospective randomized multicenter trial of empirical antitachycardia pacing versus shocks for spontaneous rapid ventricular tachycardia in patients with implantable cardioverter-defibrillators: Pacing Fast Ventricular Tachycardia Reduces Shock Therapies (PainFREE Rx II) trial results. Circulation 2004;110:2591–6.

16. Larsen GK, Evans J, Lambert WE, et al. Shocks burden and increased mortality in implantable cardioverter-defibrillator patients. Heart Rhythm 2011;8:1881–6.

17. Shamim W, Francis DP, Yousufuddin M, et al. Intraventricular conduction delay: a prognostic marker in chronic heart failure. Int J Cardiol 1999;70:171–8.

18. Kirk JA, Kass DA. Electromechanical dyssynchrony and resynchronization of the failing heart. Circ Res 2013;113:765–76.

19. Kirk JA, Kass DA. Cellular and molecular aspects of dyssynchrony and resynchronization. Heart Fail Clin 2017;13:29–41.

20. Abraham WT. Cardiac resynchronization therapy for heart failure: biventricular pacing and beyond. Curr Opin Cardiol 2002;17:346–52.

21. Wells G, Parkash R, Healey JS, et al. Cardiac resynchronization therapy: a meta-analysis of randomized controlled trials. CMAJ 2011;183:421–9.

22. Tracy CM, Epstein AE, Darbar D, et al. 2012 ACCF/AHA/HRS Focused Update of the 2008 Guidelines for Device-Based Therapy of Cardiac Rhythm Abnormalities: a report of the American College of Cardiology Foundation/American Heart Association Task Force on Practice Guidelines. Heart Rhythm 2012;9:1737–53.

23. Forleo GB, Santini L, Giammaria M, et al. Multipoint pacing via a quadripolar left-ventricular lead: preliminary results from the Italian registry on multipoint left-ventricular pacing in cardiac resynchronization therapy (IRON-MPP). Europace 2017;19:1170–7.

24. Occhetta E, Bortnik M, Magnani A, et al. Prevention of ventricular desynchronization by permanent para-Hisian pacing after atrioventricular node ablation in chronic atrial fibrillation: a crossover, blinded, randomized study versus apical right ventricular pacing. J Am Coll Cardiol 2006;47:1938–45.

25. Sharma PS, Dandamudi G, Herweg B, et al. Permanent His-bundle pacing as an alternative to biventricular pacing for cardiac resynchronization therapy: a multicenter experience. Heart Rhythm 2018;15:413–20.

26. de Oliveira JC, Martinelli M, Nishioka SA, et al. Efficacy of antibiotic prophylaxis before the implantation of pacemakers and cardioverter-defibrillators: results of a

large, prospective, randomized, double-blinded, placebo-controlled trial. Circ Arrhythm Electrophysiol 2009;2:29–34.

27. Baddour LM, Epstein AE, Erickson CC, et al. Update on cardiovascular implantable electronic device infections and their management: a scientific statement from the American Heart Association. Circulation 2010;121:458–77.

28. Wilkoff BL, Auricchio A, Brugada J, et al. HRS/EHRA Expert Consensus on the Monitoring of Cardiovascular Implantable Electronic Devices (CIEDs): description of techniques, indications, personnel, frequency and ethical considerations: developed in partnership with the Heart Rhythm Society (HRS) and the European Heart Rhythm Association (EHRA); and in collaboration with the American College of Cardiology (ACC), the American Heart Association (AHA), the European Society of Cardiology (ESC), the Heart Failure Association of ESC (HFA), and the Heart Failure Society of America (HFSA). Endorsed by the Heart Rhythm Society, the European Heart Rhythm Association (a registered branch of the ESC), the American College of Cardiology, the American Heart Association. Europace 2008;10:707–25.

29. Lampert R, Hayes DL, Annas GJ, et al. HRS Expert Consensus Statement on the Management of Cardiovascular Implantable Electronic Devices (CIEDs) in patients nearing end of life or requesting withdrawal of therapy. Heart Rhythm 2010;7:1008–26.

30. Indik JH, Gimbel JR, Abe H, et al. 2017 HRS expert consensus statement on magnetic resonance imaging and radiation exposure in patients with cardiovascular implantable electronic devices. Heart Rhythm 2017;14:e97–153.

31. Hayes DL, Asirvatham SJ, Freedman PA. Cardiac pacing, defibrillation and resynchronization: a clinical approach. 3rd edition. West Sussex (United Kingdom): Wiley-Backwell; 2013.

Arrhythmias in Congenital Heart Disease

Jessica Kline, DO[a], Otto Costantini, MD[b],*

KEYWORDS

- Congenital heart disease • Arrhythmias • Atrial arrhythmia • Ventricular arrhythmia

KEY POINTS

- Cardiac defects are the most common congenital defects, accounting for approximately 9 per 1000 births.
- Patients with structural heart disease related to congenital diseases are prone to develop intrinsic rhythm abnormalities as a result of altered physiology. In addition, they are at an increased risk of developing acquired arrhythmias secondary to the nature of surgical interventions done to improve physiologic function in the setting of these defects.
- Arrhythmia management and risk stratification poses a particularly complex challenge to clinicians managing this population.

INTRODUCTION

Nearly one-third of all major congenital anomalies are cardiac defects affecting approximately 9 per 1000 births worldwide.[1] Most importantly, due to the evolution of surgical interventions, many patients born with congenital heart defects are living into adulthood.[2] As this population continues to age, more adults are now living with congenital heart disease (CHD) than children, accounting for approximately 3 million patients worldwide.[3]

Patients with many congenital heart abnormalities are predisposed to atrial and ventricular arrhythmias due to their structural heart disease and the anatomically abnormal conduction system and conduction tissue that is associated with the structural dysfunction. In addition, many of the surgical repairs required to fix the structural abnormalities lead to the creation of the electrophysiological substrate that results in early perioperative or late postoperative arrhythmias. Residual hemodynamic abnormalities, caused by both the intrinsic congenital defects and those acquired after the surgical corrections, predispose patients to atrial and ventricular arrhythmias.

Disclosure Statement: The authors have no financial relationships to disclose pertaining to the content of this article.

[a] Summa Health Heart & Vascular Institute, Summa Health System, 95 Arch Street, Suite 300, Akron, OH 44304, USA; [b] Cardiovascular Disease Fellowship, Summa Health Heart & Vascular Institute, Summa Health System, 95 Arch Street, Suite 350, Akron, OH 44304, USA
* Corresponding author.
E-mail address: costantinio@summahealth.org

Arrhythmia management and primary risk stratification pose particular challenges in this population because the available data are limited. The Pediatric and Congenital Electrophysiology Society (PACES) and Heart and Rhythm Society (HRS) released an expert consensus statement in 2014 that details specific recommendations for hemodynamic and electrophysiological diagnostic workups and for the use of pharmacologic, device, and ablative therapies.

ATRIAL TACHYARRHYTHMIAS
Accessory Pathway–Mediated Tachyarrhythmias or Concealed Pathway Tachyarrhythmias

Accessory pathway–mediated tachyarrhythmias or concealed pathway tachyarrhythmias are caused by anomalous bundles of conducting tissue between the atrial and ventricular myocardium that conduct outside of the normal specialized conduction system. These pathways are a result of a failure of resorption of the myocardial syncytium of the atrioventricular (AV) valves during fetal development. This tissue usually conducts faster than the AV node and, therefore, allows conduction to bypass the conduction system of the heart.

The most commonly encountered accessory pathway is associated with the bundle of Kent and leads to the Wolff-Parkinson (WPW) syndrome. It is especially common in levotransposition of the great arteries (L-TGA; congenitally corrected transposition), Ebstein anomaly, AV septal defect, and hypertrophic cardiomyopathy. WPW syndrome has the only accessory pathway that can conduct antegrade, thus, if rapid conduction is present during atrial fibrillation, ventricular fibrillation and sudden cardiac death can ensue. Concealed pathways are hidden during sinus rhythm and can only conduct retrograde.

An electrophysiology study can be used to locate the site of these accessory or concealed pathways and determine the refractory period and the likelihood that the pathway characteristics could lead to lethal arrhythmias.

Atrial Flutter (Typical Isthmus-Dependent and Atypical)

Atrial flutter is the most common arrhythmia of patients with simple or complex CHD. It occurs intrinsically in unoperated or preoperative hearts, as well as in postsurgical repair patients. The atrial flutters that occur preoperatively are a result of right atrial enlargement, which results from any single ventricle physiology or any valve disorder that leads to atrial dilatation. **Box 1** demonstrates the specific congenital heart defects.

Box 1
Specific congenital heart defects that commonly lead to preoperative atrial flutter

Atrial septal defects

AV canal defects

Total anomalous pulmonary venous connection

Tricuspid atresia

Pulmonary atresia

Mitral atresia

Aortic atresia

Tricuspid stenosis

Double-inlet single left ventricle

Double-outlet right ventricle

Patients with CHD often do not have typical isthmus-dependent atrial flutter. Instead, they have variable atrial rates. In postoperative patients, there are many different circuits that occur between suture lines and scars. Owing to variable ventricular rates, these may be confused for atrial fibrillation or atrial tachycardia. Typically, the electrocardiogram (ECG) does not have consistent atrial flutter waves. These circuits can occur after any surgical procedure involving the atrium. They are more difficult to define and ablate than typical atrial flutter and are complex intraatrial reentrant tachycardias (IARTs).

Intraatrial Reentrant Tachyarrhythmias

IARTs are macroreentrant tachyarrhythmias that do not involve the cavotricuspid valve isthmus as typical atrial flutter does. They occur after atrial septal defect (ASD) repairs, Mustard and Senning procedures,[4] Fontan palliative repair, and repair of anomalous pulmonary venous return. They are more likely to occur in ASD correction that occurs at a later age.[5] These arrhythmias are hemodynamically detrimental owing to the loss of AV synchrony. They also cause increased atrial thrombosis, which can be catastrophic. Similar to intrinsic atrial flutter, they tend to have a slower atrial rate and thus a typically a slower ventricular rate that could be mistaken for sinus rhythm.

Symptoms and presentation depend on the hemodynamic effects. Patients may be asymptomatic, or present with dyspnea, palpitations, lightheadedness, or (more rarely) syncope. The ECG can be difficult to discern from sinus tachycardia or from a focal atrial tachycardia; however, clinicians should have a high index of suspicion in patients with history of surgery.

Atrial Fibrillation

Atrial fibrillation may occur in up to 30% of patients with congenital heart defects. Like atrial flutter, it occurs in defects that result in high atrial pressure, subsequent volume overload, and atrial dilatation.[6]

VENTRICULAR TACHYARRHYTHMIAS
Junctional Tachyarrhythmia (Junctional Ectopic or His Bundle Tachycardia)

Junctional ectopic tachyarrhythmia is a ventricular tachyarrhythmia that typically occurs in the first 24 to 72 hours following repair of specific congenital heart defects (**Box 2**). The exact pathophysiology is not known but it is thought to be due to postoperative inflammation, hypoxia, or direct surgical trauma. It is a narrow-complex tachycardia that occurs at greater than 200 beats per minute, with ventriculoatrial dissociation that is life-threatening. The high mortality rate is a result of acute cardiogenic shock and low cardiac output if the rhythm cannot be stopped.[7]

Box 2
Postoperative congenital heart disease most at risk for junctional ectopic tachycardia

Tetralogy of Fallot (ventricular septal defect [VSD] repair)

Dextrotransposition of the great arteries (Mustard and Senning procedure)

VSD closure

Total anomalous venous return

Single ventricle physiology (Fontan procedure)

Direct current cardioversion is not useful because, typically, the arrhythmia will quickly return. The goal of acute treatment is to slow the ventricular rate to less than 150 beats per minute. Pharmacotherapy can include class I antiarrhythmic therapy, including flecainide and propafenone, and class III antiarrhythmic amiodarone.[8]

BRADYARRHYTHMIAS
Sinus Node Dysfunction

Sinus node dysfunction can be either intrinsic or acquired as an early or late postoperative complication. The suggested pathophysiology is progressive fibrosis of the sinoatrial tissue either after surgery or the long-term hemodynamic compromise from the congenital heart defect. It can occur in any surgical operation but especially in those with extensive atrial repair, such as Mustard, Senning, Glenn, Fontan, and Ebstein procedures. It is suggested that 90% of post-Mustard operation patients will have sinus node dysfunction within 10 years of the procedure and that approximately 10% to 20% will require permanent pacemaker placement.[9,10] It can also occur after repair of superior sinus venosus defects owing to the proximity to the sinus node,[11] and with heterotaxy and juxtaposed atrial appendage patients.[12]

Patients will present with dizziness and lightheadedness or symptoms of chronotropic incompetence such as fatigue. Further morbidity and progression of symptoms can result from the loss of AV synchrony, causing low ventricular function due to slow rates.

Atrioventricular Node Dysfunction or Atrioventricular Block

The AV node is located at the base of the right atrium and is found in the center of the Koch triangle, of which the boundaries are the septal leaflet of the tricuspid valve, the coronary sinus, and the membranous part of the interatrial septum.[13] In the acute postoperative setting, AV block occurs with defects and procedures that are near the AV node. These include ventricular septal defect (VSD) closures, especially the perimembranous ventricular septum; AV septal defects; repair of the aortic valve; or subaortic stenosis procedures.

The American Heart Association guidelines recommend permanent pacing if the AV block has not recovered within 7 to 9 days of surgery.[14] Despite recovery, patients may develop late AV block up to 10 to 15 years postoperatively, especially after AV septal repairs. Weindling and colleagues[15] found that, although 90% of patients recover from AV conduction within 9 days, in the long-term the incidence of death is at least 60%. Therefore, they recommend pacemaker placement in all patients.

Congenital Atrioventricular Block

Congenital AV block has variable presentation. Some patients are diagnosed in utero owing to low fetal heart rates. Other children will be asymptomatic and later develop heart failure and eventual cardiac collapse if undetected. AV block is associated with L-TGA and heterotaxy syndromes.

ARRHYTHMIAS OF SPECIFIC CONGENITAL HEART DEFECTS
Complete (Dextrotransposition) of the Great Arteries

Dextrotransposition of the great arteries (D-TGA) describes complete transposition of the 2 main arteries: the aorta and the pulmonary artery. The aorta typically overlies the pulmonary artery; however, in the case of D-TGA, the aorta lies behind the pulmonary artery. In this congenital abnormality, oxygen-rich blood is continuously pumped from the left ventricle to the pulmonary artery and back to the lungs. The oxygen-depleted blood is pumped from the right ventricle through the aorta, then to the rest of the body. Patients depend on the presence of an ASD or VSD to allow for mixing of oxygenated blood and require surgery right after birth.

The Mustard and Senning procedures were developed to redirect venous caval blood flow to the left atrium and left ventricle to allow for oxygenation. The techniques are similar and primarily differ in the material used to create a conduit to the left atrium. These techniques were used up until the early 1980s when advancements in cardiopulmonary bypass allowed for arterial switch procedures. They both require extensive atriotomy and atrial surgery and use the right ventricle as the systemic ventricle, with significant long-term hemodynamic implications. Ventricular tachycardia (VT) can occur years after the procedures as a result of long-standing right ventricular dysfunction.

Patients have greater than 50% incidence of atrial arrhythmias, including bradyarrhythmias and ectopic atrial rhythms. They are a direct result of intraoperative damage to the sinus node, sinus node artery, intranodal pathways, or the AV node itself. Up to 25% of patients will require a pacemaker. Patients have a 2% to 10% risk of sudden death most likely related to 1:1 intraatrial reentrant tachyarrhythmias that lead to ventricular fibrillation, asystole, or electromechanical dissociation.[16] Predictors of sudden cardiac death include older age at time of repair, abnormal hemodynamics, development of atrial flutter or IART, sick sinus syndrome, and ventricular arrhythmias.[17,18] Owing to these extensive complications, the arterial switch procedure has largely replaced the Mustard and Senning operations and has not shown evidence of arrhythmias since its adoption in the mid-1980s.

Single Ventricle

The single ventricle physiology is a complex defect due to a single functional ventricle, the lack of a heart valve, or an abnormality in the pumping function of a ventricle. It is surgically palliated via the Fontan procedure, which redirects venous caval blood directly to the pulmonary arteries. Patients usually have this procedure around 2 to 5 years of age as the final procedure in a series of 3 procedures.

Similar to patients who have the Mustard and Senning procedures, patients who undergo extensive intraatrial surgery are at risk for supraventricular tachycardias and bradyarrhythmias due to sinus node dysfunction, and have a long-standing risk for VT due to poor long-term hemodynamics (**Table 1**).

Table 1	
Arrhythmias associated with single ventricle physiology and their incidence	
Sinus node dysfunction	15%–50%
AV block	9.5%
Junctional rhythm	8%
Atrial flutter or IART	42%–57%
Ectopic atrial rhythm	19%
Junctional ectopic tachycardia	48%
VT	7.5%
Sudden cardiac death	3%

Data from Ghai A, Harris L, Harrison DA, et al. Outcomes of late atrial tachyarrhythmias in adults after the Fontan operation. J Am Coll Cardiol 2001;37(2):585–592; and van den Bosch AE, Roos-Hesselink JW, Van Domburg R, et al. Long-term outcome and quality of life in adult patients after the Fontan operation. Am J Cardiol 2004;93(9):1141–1145.

Junctional ectopic tachycardia is a life-threatening arrhythmia that occurs in the early postoperative period in about 10% to 15% of patients.[19] This is thought to be secondary to the chronic high atrial pressure. Late arrhythmias include bradyarrhythmias, likely a direct cause of progressive sinus node fibrosis or direct surgical disruption. Atrial flutter, IART, ectopic atrial tachycardia, ventricular arrhythmias, and sudden death are due to the long-standing volume overload, ventricular hypertrophy, and fibrosis. Surgical modifications, including extracardiac conduits and lateral tunnel techniques, have decreased the amount of intraatrial surgery and reduced the chronic high atrial pressures, thus leading to fewer arrhythmias.[20–22]

Ebstein Anomaly

Ebstein anomaly is the downward displacement of the posterior and septal leaflets of the tricuspid valve toward the apex of the right ventricle. The right ventricle is, therefore, functioning as the right atrium, though morphologically and electrically it remains the right ventricle. Thus, when arrhythmias develop, they are not well-tolerated owing to the already compromised hemodynamics.

The atrial arrhythmia predominantly associated with this defect is an accessory pathway–mediated tachycardia (WPW syndrome). Accessory pathways are almost always right-sided and occur in up to 25% of patients with Ebstein anomaly.[23] When an accessory pathway is present, the typical right bundle branch block that is present on the ECG of patients with Ebstein may be absent. Other atrial tachyarrhythmias, such as atrial flutter and atrial fibrillation, may occur due to a large right atrium and high right atrial pressures. These are not typically seen until the patients are greater than 35 years old.

Before surgical repair, all patients should undergo an electrophysiology study to characterize the accessory pathway. During surgery, they should undergo a right-sided maze or cryoablation procedure to decrease the long-term risk of IART and sudden cardiac death.

Tetralogy of Fallot

Tetralogy of Fallot (TOF) is characterized by 4 defects: a VSD, an overriding aorta, pulmonary stenosis, and right ventricular hypertrophy. Pulmonary stenosis occurs due to malalignment of the infundibulum of the right ventricular outflow tract with subsequent tricuspid stenosis. Surgical repair includes a patch closure of the VSD with the resection of a large part of the right ventricle. A large transannular patch of the pulmonary valve annulus is constructed to relieve the right ventricular outflow tract stenosis.

These surgical repairs cause chronic cyanosis, which is responsible for progressive ventricular fibrosis due to wall stress from volume overload. After repair, atrial arrhythmias occur in approximately one-third of adult patients and are an independent risk factor for sudden cardiac death. They are more common in the presence of pulmonary regurgitation, left ventricular dysfunction, and high right atrial volume.[24] VT occurs in 30% of patients and is associated with several risk factors depicted (**Box 3**). Pulmonary valve replacement seems to decrease episodes of VT and atrial flutter, likely due to decreased volume and pressure overload.[25]

Atrial Septal Defect

ASD occurs as a result of incomplete septation of the atria during the embryonic development of the heart. There are 4 different types of ASD, each associated with different rhythm disturbances. If left unrepaired, an ASD can result in Eisenmenger syndrome, the volume overload of the right atrium due to the left-to-right shunting. This causes a high burden of atrial fibrillation and other atrial tachyarrhythmias.

Box 3
Risk factors for ventricular tachycardia after tetralogy of Fallot repair

General risk factors

Older age at repair

Long postoperative repair period

Right ventricular systolic pressure greater than 60 mm Hg at rest

Decreased left ventricular function

Moderate to severe pulmonary or tricuspid regurgitation

Increased right ventricular end-diastolic volume

Right ventricular diastolic pressure greater than 10 mm Hg

ECG risk factors

QRS greater than 180 ms

Rate of change of QRS greater than 3.5–4 ms/y

QRS, QTc, or JTc dispersion

Signal-averaged ECG with late potentials

Inducible monomorphic or polymorphic VT

ASDs affect the conduction system directly by causing inferior-posterior displacement of the AV node, left bundle branch block, and relative hypoplasia of the anterior portion of the left bundle, causing left axis deviation. If an ASD occurs in the setting of a large AV septal defect, accessory AV pathways are typically found in the posteroseptal region, leading to accessory pathway–mediated tachyarrhythmias. With an ostium secundum ASD or a sinus venosus repair, bradyarrhythmias can occur due to direct damage to the sinus node or AV node.

Ventricular Septal Defect

VSDs are the most common congenital cardiac defect.[26] They can occur anywhere within the interventricular septum. Regardless of location, arrhythmias are common and a result of hemodynamic changes from increased pulmonary artery pressures, similar to that seen in TOF patients. The incidence of sudden cardiac death is less than 5% and typically associated with increased pulmonary vascular resistance, surgery occurring later than 5 years old, or untreated heart block due to ventricular hypertrophy and conduction system fibrosis.

DIAGNOSIS AND MONITORING

Patients with congenital heart defects, whether simplex or complex, should be monitored for arrhythmias on a regular basis. The PACES-HRS expert consensus statement on arrhythmias in adult CHD developed recommendations regarding monitoring, diagnosis, and treatment based on expert opinion and available data.[27]

The definition of simple, moderate, and complex CHD found in the expert consensus guidelines are beyond the scope of this article. However, patients with complex or moderately complex CHD should be followed yearly with routine ECG and hemodynamic echo assessments. Those with simple CHD should be followed occasionally with such assessments, though exactly how often remains unclear. Patients with implanted cardiac rhythm monitoring devices should have routine interrogations as per standard care. Exercise stress testing is often routinely initiated at puberty to assess for symptoms of arrhythmia, syncope, exercise-induced arrhythmias, and exercise tolerance, and to evaluate chronotropic competence, especially in those with complex CHD.

If a patient presents with symptoms suggestive of an arrhythmia, such as palpitation, dizziness, or syncope, they should undergo a thorough history, physical examination, 12-lead ECG, and 24-hour or 30-day ambulatory ECG monitoring if the symptoms are sporadic. If these tests are unrevealing but a high index of clinical suspicion remains, then patients should receive an implantable loop recorder. An echocardiogram for hemodynamic assessment should also be done. If the images are poor, they should be imaged with a computed tomography scan or MRI. A patient who presents with unexplained syncope or has high-risk CHD substrates should undergo an electrophysiological study. This includes patients with TOF, D-TGA status/post arterial switch, ventricular dysfunction, or single ventricle physiology.

MANAGEMENT
Atrial Arrhythmias

If the patient is hemodynamically stable, the goal in atrial tachyarrhythmias is rate control. However, given that many CHD patients have tenuous hemodynamic function to begin with, these rhythms are often not well-tolerated. Direct current cardioversion is the preferred option in the acute setting if the patient is hemodynamically unstable. Specifically, IART typically has a slow cycle length and can change among different pathways, causing variable ventricular rates. These patients should be cardioverted to sinus rhythm because they have a 20% incidence of sudden cardiac death if they remain in IART. Longer term treatment options will vary by patient, depending on coexisting comorbidities, including sinus node dysfunction, impaired AV nodal conduction, ventricular dysfunction, and their childbearing potential.

Oral anticoagulation or thrombolysis

Recommendations regarding oral anticoagulation are the same as standard recommendations. If the patient's atrial tachyarrhythmia is greater than 48 hours or of unknown duration, a transesophageal echo-guided cardioversion or oral anticoagulation for 3 weeks before cardioversion are indicated. Anticoagulation is indicated in patients who have complex congenital heart defects, sustained or recurrent IART, or atrial fibrillation. Such patients have a higher than expected risk for thromboembolic complications. The ChADS$_2$VASC scoring for the risk of thromboembolism should not be used in CHD patients because it is not applicable.[28] Direct oral anticoagulants have not been well-studied in these patients but initial data are promising in patients who do not have prosthetic valves.[29] A vitamin K antagonist is the most commonly used and most studied agent. It should be noted that these patients have several factors that increase their bleeding risk, including liver dysfunction, renal dysfunction, and chronic cyanosis.

Pharmacotherapy

Antiarrhythmic agent options are limited by multiple organ comorbidities that make the use of these drugs challenging. Amiodarone is often the first-line treatment owing to lack of alternative options, especially for patients who have pathologic hypertrophy and ventricular dysfunction. However, it also should be avoided in patients with hepatic, pulmonary, or thyroid disease. It should not be used in those with cyanotic heart defect, low body mass index, or prolonged QT interval greater than 460 ms or greater than 500 ms if underlying conduction disease is present. This can be problematic because many complex CHD patients have many of these comorbidities. Dofetilide is a viable alternative in patients with creatinine clearance greater than 20 mL/min, no hypokalemia, and with a QTc interval less than 440 ms or less than 500 ms if underlying conduction disease is present. In patients with simple CHD, any therapy can be considered safe and a rate-controlling strategy may be more successful.

Catheter ablation

Catheter ablation options have expanded as more advanced mapping techniques have become available and access to complex structures is more feasible. The most important aspect of successful and safe ablation is an advanced understanding of the anatomy, prior surgical repair, and the use of 3-dimensional mapping technology.[30] Patients with CHD have thicker atrial tissue, which has required development of irrigated ablation catheters and larger tips.[31] Due to the complexities of this tissue, ablations are less successful, with recurrence rates of approximately 40%.[32] Because it is well-established that atrial tachyarrhythmias increase the risk of sudden death, ablation is still the treatment of choice for patients who are symptomatic and refractory to antiarrhythmic therapy. Patients with ventricular preexcitation (WPW syndrome) or with high-risk or multiple accessory pathways should be strongly considered for ablative therapy. Finally, as a last resort, AV nodal ablation and permanent pacemaker placement is an option.

Surgical prescription

There are no surgical procedures that have proven beneficial in decreasing arrhythmias. However, modern modifications of surgical techniques have made arrhythmias less likely to occur. For example, in the case of atrial tachyarrhythmias, the use of lateral tunnel techniques, the utilization of extracardiac conduits, and the overall decrease of atrial scar tissue have proven most successful. Other surgical techniques include the creation of anchoring lesions between surgical scars and key anatomic boundaries with cryoablation. The PACES-HRS guidelines recommend that patients with documented atrial arrhythmias before surgery should undergo a surgical maze procedure with or without cavotricuspid isthmus ablation at the time of surgery.

Ventricular Arrhythmias

Patients uncommonly present with sustained ventricular tachyarrhythmias.[33] However, VT is not well-tolerated and should be treated as an emergency. Underlying extracardiac causes, such as electrolyte abnormalities, hypoxia, or acidosis, should be corrected. VT is most commonly seen in patients with TOF or CHD with long-standing increased ventricular pressure, such as aortic stenosis, single ventricle physiology, complete transposition, or abnormal myocardium due to fibrosis or hypertrophy.

Acute treatment

Lidocaine bolus and continuous drip should be the first-line pharmacotherapy for VT, with careful monitoring of lidocaine concentration to prevent toxicity. Synchronized cardioversion at 2 to 5 J/kg is the next step when pharmacotherapy fails or if patient is hemodynamically unstable or lacks intravenous access. Occasionally, rapid ventricular pacing can also be used to attempt conversion.

Chronic treatment

If patients have VT in the early postoperative period, they are more likely to have a late presentation of VT. Patients should undergo regular thorough investigation of hemodynamic abnormalities, usually by noninvasive means, including echocardiography. These patients often require chronic drug regimens. The PACES-HRS guidelines recommend that if patients remain refractory to pharmacotherapy they should have implantation of a cardioverter-defibrillator.

Catheter ablation
Patients with life-threatening VT refractory to drugs or device therapy, or those with frequent ventricular ectopy resulting in decreased ventricular function, may require electrophysiological study with catheter-based ablation to at least decrease the episodes. Patients with TOF should have specific anatomic sites ablated for higher success rates.[34] Ablation therapy is not appropriate as a prophylactic therapy for sudden death because it has not been shown to reduce the risk.

Bradyarrhythmias

Device use
Bradyarrhythmias requiring permanent pacemaker placement are highly prevalent in patients with CHD. Some CHD may cause bradyarrhythmias at birth but most bradyarrhythmias occur after surgical intervention. As previously discussed, advancements in surgical techniques and avoidance of causing damage to conducting tissue have helped to improve the incidence postoperatively. If permanent pacemaker placement is required, an electrophysiologist with expertise in CHD should be consulted. Permanent pacemaker placement is often complicated by obstructed venous access and difficult anatomic considerations for lead placement that can lead to high rates of complications. When patients require permanent pacing, they are typically pacemaker-dependent, thus clinicians must be diligent in surveillance of the device. They should be monitored for wire fracture, impedance changes, or threshold changes.

SUDDEN CARDIAC DEATH

The sudden cardiac death rate of patients with CHD is 25 to 100 times higher than that of the general population.[35] However, the incidence of sudden death remains relatively low. It seems to be highest for cyanotic lesion, such as TOF and dextrotransposition, and for aortic obstructive lesions, such as aortic stenosis and coarctation of the aorta. In such patients, the risk may be as high as 10% to 15% after 20 to 25 years of follow-up. Specific risk factors include residual hemodynamic dysfunction, late surgical repair, age greater than 25 years after surgical repair, QRS greater than 180 ms, nonsustained VT, right ventricular outflow tract patch, and ECG consistent with dispersion of repolarization. Risk stratification has been a particularly difficult topic. Many congenital cardiac defects have not been extensively studied or followed long-term and the true risk is not known.[36] The utility of an electrophysiology study for inducible ventricular arrhythmias is unclear; however, if a ventricular arrhythmia can be induced, this is an independent risk factor and patients should undergo implantable cardioverter-defibrillator placement. Risk stratification should be combined with sound clinical judgment by those with expertise in CHD.

REFERENCES

1. Van der Linde D, Konings EE, Slager MA, et al. Birth prevalence of congenital heart disease worldwide: review and meta-analyses. J Am Coll Cardiol 2011; 58:2241-7.

2. Khairy P, Ionescu-Htu R, Mackie AS, et al. Changing mortality in congenital heart disease. J Am Coll Cardiol 2010;56:1149–57.
3. Marelli AJ, Mackie AS, Ionescu-Htu R, et al. Congenital heart disease in the general population: changing prevalence and age distribution. Circulation 2007;115: 163–72.
4. Gewillig M, Wyse RK, de Leval MR, et al. Early and late arrhythmias after the Fontan operation: predisposing factors and clinical consequences. Br Heart J 1992; 67:72–9.
5. Gatzoulis MA, Freeman MA, Siu SC, et al. Atrial arrhythmia after surgical closure of atrial septal defects in adults. N Engl J Med 1999;340:839–46.
6. Kirsh JA, Walsh EP, Triedman JK. Prevalence of and risk factors for atrial fibrillation and intra-atrial re-entrant tachycardia among patients with congenital heart disease. Am J Cardiol 2002;90(3):338.
7. Rhodes LA, Walsh EP, Gamble WJ, et al. Benefits and potential risks of atrial anti-tachycardia pacing after repair of congenital heart disease. Pacing Clin Electrophysiol 1995;18:1005–16.
8. Walsh EP, Saul JP, Sholler GF, et al. Evaluation of a staged treatment protocol for rapid automatic junctional tachycardia after operation for congenital heart disease. J Am Coll Cardiol 1997;29:1046–55.
9. Lange R, Horer J, Kostolny M, et al. Presence of a ventricular septal defect and the Mustard operation are risk factors for late mortality after the atrial switch operation: thirty years of follow-up in 417 patients at a single center. Circulation 2006; 114:1905–13.
10. Moons P, Gewillig M, Sluysmans T, et al. Long term outcome up to 30 years after the Mustard or Senning operation: a nationwide multicentre study in Belgium. Heart 2004;90:307–13.
11. Oliver JM, Gallego P, Gonzalez A, et al. Sinus venosus syndrome: atrial septal defect or anomalous venous connection? A multiplan transesophageal approach. Heart 2002;88(6):634–8.
12. Anjos RT, Ho SY, Anderson RH. Surgical implications of juxtaposition of the atrial appendages. A review of forty-nine autopsied hearts. J Thorac Cardiovasc Surg 1990;999(5):897.
13. Harrison's Principles of Internal Medicine, 17e. Section 3: disorders of rhythm.
14. Epstein AE, DiMarco JP, Ellenbogen KA, et al. ACC/AHA/HRS 2008 guidelines for device-based therapy of cardiac rhythm abnormalities. J Am Coll Cardiol 2008; 51:2085–105.
15. Weindling SN, Saul JP, Gamble WJ, et al. Duration of complete atrioventricular block after congenital heart disease surgery. Am J Cardiol 1998;82:525–7.
16. Vetter VL. Postoperative pediatric electrocardiographic and electrophysiologic sequelae. In: Liebman J, Plonsey R, Rudy Y, editors. Pediatric and fundamental electrocardiography. Boston: Martinus Nijhoff; 1987. p. 187–206.
17. Vetter VL, Tanner CS, Horowitz LN. Inducible atrial flutter after the Mustard repair of complete transposition of the great arteries. Am J Cardiol 1988;61:428–35.
18. Garson A, Bink-Boelkens M, Hesslein PS. Atrial flutter in the young: a collaborative study of 380 cases. J Am Coll Cardiol 1985;6:871–8.
19. Chen SC, Nouri S, Pennington DG. Dysrhythmias after the modified Fontan procedure. Pediatr Cardiol 1988;9:215–9.
20. Kreutzer J, Keane JF, Lock JE, et al. Conversion of modified Fontan procedure to lateral atrial tunnel cavopulmonary anastomosis. J Thorac Cardiovasc Surg 1996; 111:1169–76.

21. Sheikh AM, Tang AT, Roman K, et al. The failing Fontan circulation: successful conversion of atriopulmonary connections. J Thorac Cardiovasc Surg 2004; 128:60–6.
22. Nurnberg JH, Ovroutski S, Alexi-Meskishvili V, et al. New onset arrhythmias after the extracardiac conduit Fontan operation compared with the intraatrial lateral tunnel procedure: early and midterm results. Ann Thorac Surg 2004;78:1979–88.
23. Van Hare GF. Radiofrequency ablation of accessory pathways associated with congenital heart disease. Pacing Clin Electrophysiol 1997;20:2077–81.
24. Gatzoulis MA, Balaji S, Webber SA, et al. Risk factors in arrhythmia and sudden cardiac death late after repair of tetralogy of Fallot: a multicenter study. Lancet 2000;356:975–81.
25. Therrien J, Siu SC, Harris L, et al. Impact of pulmonary valve replacement on arrhythmia propensity later after repair of tetralogy of Fallot. Circulation 2001; 103:2489–94.
26. Hoffman JE, Kaplan S. The incidence of congenital heart disease. J Am Coll Cardiol 2002;39:1890–900.
27. Khairy P, Van Hare G, Balaji S, et al. PACES/HRS expert consensus statement on the recognition and management of arrhythmias in adult congenital heart disease. Heart Rhythm 2014;11:e81–101.
28. Khairy P, Aboulhosn J, Broberg CS, et al. Thromboprophylaxis for atrial arrhythmias in congenital heart disease: a multicenter study. Int J Cardiol 2016;223: 729–35.
29. Pujol C, Niesert AC, Engelhardt A, et al. Usefulness of direct oral anticoagulants in adult congenital heart disease. Am J Cardiol 2016;117(3):450–5.
30. Triedman JK, Alexander ME, Love BA, et al. Influence of patient factors and ablative technologies on outcomes of radiofrequency ablation of intra-atrial re-entrant tachycardia in patients with congenital heart disease. J Am Coll Cardiol 2002;39: 1827–35.
31. Triedman JK, Saul JP, Weindling SN, et al. Radiofrequency ablation of intra-atrial reentrant tachycardia after surgical palliation of congenital heart disease. Circulation 1995;91:707–14.
32. Kannankeril PJ, Anderson ME, Rottman JN, et al. Frequency of late recurrence of intra-atrial reentry tachycardia after radiofrequency catheter ablation in patients with congenital heart disease. Am J Cardiol 2003;92:879–81.
33. Koyak Z, Harris L, de Groot JR, et al. Sudden cardiac death in adult congenital heart disease. Circulation 2012;126(16):1944–54.
34. Zeppenfeld K, Schalij MJ, Bartelings MM, et al. Catheter ablation of ventricular tachycardia after repair of congenital heart disease: electroanatomic identification of the critical right ventricular isthmus. Circulation 2007;116:2241–52.
35. Silka mJ, Hardy BG, Menashe VD, et al. A population-based prospective evaluation of risk of sudden cardiac death after operation for common congenital heart defects. J Am Coll Cardiol 1998;32:245–51.
36. Khairy P, Harris L, Landzberg MJ, et al. Implantable cardioverter-defibrillators in tetralogy of Fallot. Circulation 2008;117:363–70.

Printed and bound by CPI Group (UK) Ltd, Croydon, CR0 4YY

03/10/2024

01040484-0020